RECENT ADVANCES IN HEMATOLOGY RESEARCH

HISTONE DEACETYLASE INHIBITORS (HDIS)

PHARMACOLOGY, USES AND HEALTH EFFECTS

Recent Advances in Hematology Research

Additional books in this series can be found on Nova's website under the Series tab.

Additional e-books in this series can be found on Nova's website under the e-book tab.

RECENT ADVANCES IN HEMATOLOGY RESEARCH

HISTONE DEACETYLASE INHIBITORS (HDIS)

PHARMACOLOGY, USES AND HEALTH EFFECTS

BEVERLY D. CARSON
EDITOR

New York

Library of Congress Cataloging-in-Publication Data

ISBN: 978-1-63463-835-7
Library of Congress Control Number: 2015933897

Published by Nova Science Publishers, Inc. † New York

Contents

PREFACE

This book focuses on the use of HDIs for the treatment of lymphoid malignancies; myeloid malignancies; and breast cancer.

Chapter 1 - Histone deacetylase (HDAC) is a good anti-cancer target. Histone acetyltransferases (HATs) and HDACs play an opposite role in the regulation of gene expression via an epigenetic mechanism. HATs catalyze the acetylation of lysine residues in histone tails, facilitating and sustaining gene transcription. HDACs remove the acetyl moieties from the epsilon-amine of lysine residues of histone tails, lead to more condensed form of chromatin and prevent gene transcription. There are more than 18 mammalian HDAC enzymes identified to date that are classified in four groups (class I, IIa, IIb and IV for HDACs 1-11 and class III for sirtuins 1-7. The classical HDACs contain zinc catalytic binding domains and the sirtuins represent the nonmetal-dependent enzymes. HDAC inhibitors (HDACIs) have the ability to block the activities of HDACs and function as effective anti-cancer agents. HDACIs can be classified into different structural groups: the hydroxamic acids, cyclic peptides, benzamides and short-chain fatty acids. The hydroxamates include trichostatin A, vorinostat, panobinostat, belinostat, givinostat, abexinostat, resminostat and about six other compounds. The cyclic peptides include depsipeptide and trapoxin. Benzamides include entinostat, mocetinostat, N-acetyl-dinaline and chidamide. Short-chain fatty acids include butyrate, sodium phenylbutyrate, pivaloyloxymethyl butyrate and valproic acid. The hydroxamates inhibit all classes of HDACs. Other compounds are more specific. The benzamide entinostat inhibit class I HDACs and the short-chain fatty acids, butyrate and valproic acids, inhibit class I and IIa HDACs. Mocetinostat inhibits HDACs 1, 2, 3 and 11. Tubacin is selective inhibitor of HDAC6. In addition to effect on gene expression, targeting of histones by

HDACIs influences DNA replication and repair. HDACIs are also able to regulate apoptosis, cell-cycle arrest, reactive oxygen species-induced cell death, necrosis, autophagy, differentiation and migration of cells. HDAC inhibition affects the balance between pro- and anti-apoptotic proteins involved in cell death. Malignant cells treated by HDACIs showed a significant elevation in the p53 protein level, suggesting a post-transcriptional regulation. Hyperacetylation stabilizes p53 protein levels. Combination of HDACIs and proteasome inhibitors further elevated the p53 protein level and pro-apoptotic effect in malignant cells. The effect of HDACIs is relatively selective for transformed cells over normal cells. HDACIs may also have indirect effects on tumor growth by regulating the host immune response and the tumor vasculature.

Chapter 2 - Histone deacetylase inhibitors (HDACIs) are currently used in the clinic for the treatment of solid and hematological malignancies. In particular, vorinostat (Zolinza) and romidepsin (Istodax) have been approved by the US Food and Drug Administration for the treatment of relapsed and refractory cutaneous T-cell lymphomas (CTCL) patients who have received one or more prior systemic therapy and patients with peripheral T-cell lymphoma (PTCL) who have also received one or more prior therapy. CTCL is the disease with the highest clinical response rates with HDACIs.

Therefore, the studies of the molecular basis of this responsiveness were done in CTCL. At least 35 CpG islands were hypermethylated in tumor stage CTCL samples including that of the putative tumor suppressor gene BCL-7a (B-cell CLL/Lymphoma 7) in 48% of samples. BCL-7, which is located on chromosome 12q 24.31, has been cloned as part of the chromosomal translocations in Burkitt's lymphoma and is at a site of frequent breakpoints in lymphomas. Further hypermethylated genes can be grouped into cell cycle desregulation (p15, p16 and p73), defective DNA repair gene MGMT (O-6-methylguanine-DNA methyltransferase), apoptosis dysregulation (TMS1/Target of Methylation-mediated Silencing/and p73) and chromosomal instability (G2/M checkpoint regulator gene CHFR). p73 is responsible for activation of induced death of T-cells and its silencing leads to accumulation of T cells in tissues, an important step in the pathogenesis of CTCL. Hypermethylation of p73 has also been described in nodal B-cell and NK-cell lymphomas. HDACIs block cell proliferation and cause apoptosis by altering the expression of proteins (cyclins, cyclin dependent kinase inhibitors) involved in growth control.

There is increasing evidence that HDACIs also affect several pathways that are important in cell proliferation and differentiation of lymphoid cells, including the TGF beta pathway, the JAK-STAT pathway, myc and Bcl-6. HDACIs induce death of tumor cells through the induction of both the internal and external pathways of apoptosis, as well as through non-apoptotic mechanisms like autophagy. HDACIs have anti-angiogenic effects.

Presently, there are no HDACIs that are approved for the treatment of B-cell lymphomas. The clinical data of HDACIs in non-Hodgkin lymphomas, mantle cell lymphoma and diffuse large B-cell lymphoma (DLBCL), are promising. High nuclear expression of HDAC2 may play an important role in survival of DLBCL patients. Several HDAC molecules are overexpressed in T-cell and B-cell lymphoid malignancies. STAT family of transcription factors (particularly STAT3 and STAT6) are activated in Hodgkin lymphoma. STAT regulation involves phosphorylation and lysine acetylation. HDACIs could play an important role also in Hodgkin lymphoma. Combinations of HDACIs with hypomethylating agents can also influence antitumor immune responses in Hodgkin lymphoma. The anticancer effects of HDACIs require the immune system. HDACIs are under intense investigation in multiple myeloma. The pro-apoptotic and cell cycle arresting properties are the best characterized features of HDACIs. Among the pleiotropic effects of HDACIs, the proteasome system is also affected and the decreased activity of the 20S proteasome and downregulation of members of ubiquitination-proteasome pathway in multiple myeloma were shown. HDACIs also affect the bone marrow microenvironment. Combinations of HDACIs and proteasome inhibitors have synergistic anticancer effect in multiple myeloma cells.

Chapter 3 - The results of current treatment for patients with acute myeloid leukemia (AML) remain poor and there is a need for innovative strategies. Epigenetic modulation became a promising approach. A number of clinical trials have studied the safety and clinical activity of histone deacetylase (HDAC) inhibitors (HDACIs) in AML and myelodysplastic syndrome (MDS). All classes of HDACIs were used: hydroxamic acids (vorinostat and panobinostat); cyclic peptide (romidepsin); benzamides (mocetinostat and entinostat); fatty acids (valproic acid). The conclusion of these studies with HDACI as a single agent was that the best use of these compounds would be in combination with other antileukemia agents. Aberrant promoter DNA hypermethylation and histone deacetylation are reversible processes implicated in myeloid leukemogenesis. A phase 1 trial looking at romidepsin and the hypomethylating agent azacitidine for AML (ROMAZA) was opened (2013-2015) in England. This trial is for patients with newly diagnosed relapsed or refractory AML who can't have standard chemotherapy treatment. In the US the similar phase 1 trial with AR-142, the novel orally bioavailable HDACI, and decitabine is provided (2013-2015). The wild-type p53 is required for induction of cell death by azacitidine in combination with romidepsin or panobinostat. Increasing anti-leukemic activity of decitabine via AR-42-induced upregulation of miR-29b and downregulation of known miR-29b targets (transcription factor SP1, DNA methyltransferases DNMT1, DNMT3A and DNMT3B) is a novel epigenetic targeting approach in AML. The combination of vorinostat with the DNA topoisomerase inhibitor idarubicin had synergistic antileukemia effect. Combinations of vorinostat with cytosine arabinoside (cytarabine) and another DNA topoisomerase inhibitor etoposide had also potent antileukemia activity. Vorinostat induces reactive oxygen species (ROS) that results in translocation of transcription factor NRF2 (nuclear factor-erythroid-2-related factor 2) from the cytoplasm to nucleus. This in turn results in the activation of expression of anti-oxidant genes involved in overcoming of ROS pathway. Valproic acid (VPA) monotherapy inhibits the proliferation of leukemic cells regardless of the expression of p-glycoprotein and multidrug resistance associated protein 1. VPA has been more frequently studied in the combinations, specifically with all- trans retinoic acid (ATRA). VPA was also combined with both ATRA and azacitidine. Phase 1 and 2 trials with panobinostat and phase 2 study of vorinostat in patients with primary myelofibrosis and post-polycythemia vera/essential thrombocythemia myelofibrosis were associated with clinical improvement with 100% reduction palpable splenomegaly and with improvement in the degree of anemia. Gene expression profiling and epigenome studies during treatment with HDACIs are ongoing in an attempt to clarify particular patterns of gene and epigenome deregulation that is necessary for a better understanding of clinical and biochemical effects of HDACIs.

Chapter 4 - Breast tumors are believed to be organized in a cellular hierarchy with a population of cancer stem cell (CSC) driving cancer progression and resistance to conventional treatment. The discovery of CSCs provides an explanation for why cancer may be so difficult to cure, and suggests new therapeutic strategies. If these cells are the tumor root, then they are the cells to be killed. CSCs retain key stem cell properties, including self-renewal (which initiates and drives tumorigenesis) and differentiation (albeit aberrant, which contributes to cellular heterogeneity). These last months several reports suggest that HDAC inhibitors can be used to drive CSCs out of their stemness state through dysregulation of the self-renewal/differentiation balance. Using HDAC inhibitors as a differentiation therapy to treat breast cancers is a promising therapeutic approach to eradicate the breast CSC pool and improve patients care.

In: Histone Deacetylase Inhibitors (HDIs)
Editor: Beverly D. Carson ISBN: 978-1-63463-835-7

Chapter 1

CLASSIFICATION AND FUNCTION OF HISTONE DEACETYLASE INHIBITORS

Ota Fuchs
Institute of Hematology and Blood Transfusion,
Prague, Czech Republic

ABSTRACT

Histone deacetylase (HDAC) is a good anti-cancer target. Histone acetyltransferases (HATs) and HDACs play an opposite role in the regulation of gene expression via an epigenetic mechanism. HATs catalyze the acetylation of lysine residues in histone tails, facilitating and sustaining gene transcription. HDACs remove the acetyl moieties from the epsilon-amine of lysine residues of histone tails, lead to more condensed form of chromatin and prevent gene transcription. There are more than 18 mammalian HDAC enzymes identified to date that are classified in four groups (class I, IIa, IIb and IV for HDACs 1-11 and class III for sirtuins 1-7. The classical HDACs contain zinc catalytic binding domains and the sirtuins represent the nonmetal-dependent enzymes. HDAC inhibitors (HDACIs) have the ability to block the activities of HDACs and function as effective anti-cancer agents. HDACIs can be classified into different structural groups: the hydroxamic acids, cyclic peptides, benzamides and short-chain fatty acids. The hydroxamates include trichostatin A, vorinostat, panobinostat, belinostat, givinostat, abexinostat, resminostat and about six other compounds. The cyclic peptides include depsipeptide and trapoxin.

Benzamides include entinostat, mocetinostat, N-acetyl-dinaline and chidamide. Short-chain fatty acids include butyrate, sodium phenylbutyrate, pivaloyloxymethyl butyrate and valproic acid. The hydroxamates inhibit all classes of HDACs. Other compounds are more specific. The benzamide entinostat inhibit class I HDACs and the short-chain fatty acids, butyrate and valproic acids, inhibit class I and IIa HDACs. Mocetinostat inhibits HDACs 1, 2, 3 and 11. Tubacin is selective inhibitor of HDAC6. In addition to effect on gene expression, targeting of histones by HDACIs influences DNA replication and repair. HDACIs are also able to regulate apoptosis, cell-cycle arrest, reactive oxygen species-induced cell death, necrosis, autophagy, differentiation and migration of cells. HDAC inhibition affects the balance between pro- and anti-apoptotic proteins involved in cell death. Malignant cells treated by HDACIs showed a significant elevation in the p53 protein level, suggesting a post-transcriptional regulation. Hyperacetylation stabilizes p53 protein levels. Combination of HDACIs and proteasome inhibitors further elevated the p53 protein level and pro-apoptotic effect in malignant cells. The effect of HDACIs is relatively selective for transformed cells over normal cells. HDACIs may also have indirect effects on tumor growth by regulating the host immune response and the tumor vasculature.

Keywords: Acetylation, apoptosis, cell cycle, histone deacetylates, HDAC inhibitors, sirtuins

INTRODUCTION

The role of acetylation and methylation of histones in the regulation of RNA synthesis was described by Allfrey et al. [1] fifty years ago. Acetylation neutralizes the positive charge of the histone lysine residues, producing a relaxed chromatin conformation. This chromatin conformation allows the access of the transcription machinery and stimulates gene transcription [2]. However, histone deacetylation induces a condensed chromatin state that is connected with repression of the gene transcription [2]. The balance between histone acetylation and deacetylation plays an important role in the epigenetic regulation of the gene expression of tumor suppressor genes or oncogenes [3-28]. This balance is usually well regulated, but is often upset in cancer. Inhibitors of HDACs (HDACIs) are under investigation as novel anti-cancer drugs, which induce histone acetylation and modulate chromatin structure that modulates the accessibility of transcription factors to their target DNA leading to transcriptional activation of genes involved in regulation of cell cycle progression, angiogenesis and apoptosis in cancer cells. Additionally, acetylation and/or deacetylation of the non-histone proteins modify many important cell functions. HDACs are enzymes that catalyze the removal of acetyl groups from lysine residues in both histone and non-histone proteins. HDACs act as components of multiprotein complexes. They play a key role in the regulation of gene transcription and many other biological processes involving chromatin. HDACs are critically involved in cell-cycle regulation, cell proliferation, differentiation, and in the development of human cancer. As expected for vital regulators of many cellular processes, the activities of HDACs are tightly controlled and precisely regulated by multiple mechanisms. The activities of most if not all HDACs are regulated by protein-protein interactions. In addition, many HDACs are regulated by post-translational modifications as well as by subcellular localization. Less studied, but perhaps equally important, is the regulation of some HDACs by control of expression, availability of cofactors, and by proteolytic processing. A complete understanding of how HDACs are regulated will contribute not only to our overall knowledge of chromatin structure and gene control, but will offer tremendous insight into approaches for developing therapeutic HDAC inhibitors with improved specificity.

Chromatin architecture of eukaryotic cells consists of tightly packed DNA, histones, and nonhistone proteins [29, 30]. The basic organizing unit of chromatin is the nucleosome. The nucleosome core contains 147 base pairs of DNA tightly wrapped around a central histone octamer (1.65 times) containing two molecules of each of the core histones (H2A, H2B, H3, and H4). Histones are alkaline proteins that are divided into core histones and linker histones (H1 and H5). The four core histones may undergo various posttranscriptional modifications, which regulate the function of chromatin. These modifications include acetylation, phosphorylation, methylation, and ubiquitination and alter interaction of histones with DNA and nuclear proteins. The combined effect of these modifications creates the so-called "histone code", an epigenetic marketing system which regulates diverse biological processes such as gene regulation, DNA repair, and chromosome condensation.

There are currently 18 mammalian HDAC enzymes that have been identified (Table 1). These enzymes are classified into four main classes, based on their homology to yeast [31, 32]. The "classical", metal-dependent HDAC enzymes involve class I, II, and IV HDACs and the sirtuins; the nonmetal-dependent enzymes represent class III. Class III HDACs consists of seven HDACs (the sirtuins, SIRT1 to SIRT7). The sirtuins share homology to the yeast silent information regulator 2 [33] and differ from the classical HDAC enzymes, as they require the consumption of nicotinamide adenine dinucleotide to deacetylate the lysine residues [34-37]. Sirtuins are a family of proteins that have diverse roles in regulating metabolism, genome stability, cell proliferation, and survival and are implicated in mammalian aging and longevity.

Table 1. Members of the metal (Zn^{2+})-dependent HDAC enzymes

HDAC enzyme	Size (amino acid)	Chromosomal size	Localization
Class I (Rpd3)			
HDAC1	482	1p34.1	Nucleus
HDAC2	488	6q21	Nucleus
HDAC3	428	5q31.3	Nucleus
HDAC8	377	Xq13	Nucleus/cytoplasm
Class IIa (Hda 1)			
HDAC4	1084	2q37.2	Nucleus/cytoplasm
HDAC5	1122	17q21	Nucleus/cytoplasm
HDAC7	912	12q13.1	Nucleus/cytoplasm
HDAC9	1069	7p12.1	Nucleus/cytoplasm
Class IIb (Hda1)			
HDAC6	1215	Xp11.22	Cytoplasm
HDAC10	669	22q13.3	Cytoplasm
Class IV (Rpd3/Hda1)			
HDAC11	347	3p25.2	Nucleus/cytoplasm

The classical HDAC enzymes are metal-dependent as they contain zinc catalytic binding domains. Class I enzymes contain HDAC1, -2, -3, and -8 and are expressed ubiquitously and are related to the yeast RDP3 deacetylase [38]. These isotypes are usually7 expressed within the nucleus and act as transcriptional corepressors. While most class I HDACs are subunits of multiprotein nuclear complexes crucial for transcriptional repression and epigenetic landscaping, class II members regulate cytoplasmic processes or act like signal transducers trafficking between the cytoplasm and the nucleus. The class II enzymes share homology with the yeast HDAC1 and are subdivided into class IIa, consisting of HDAC4, -5, -7, and -9, and class IIb, containing HDAC6 and -10 [39]. These isotypes show tissue-specific distribution and are known to shuttle between the nucleus and cytoplasm, although histone proteins broadly represent their main target. The class IIb enzymes differ in that they primarily localize to the cytoplasm and differ structurally by containing two catalytic sites [40]. HDAC11 shares homology with the class I isotypes, but shows more tissue-specific distribution with cytoplasmic localization. As it shares relationships with both class I and class II HDACs and structural homology to yeast, it has been designated a distinct class IV [32, 41]. HDACs have more than 50 nonhistone protein substrates, such as DNA-binding proteins, transcription factors, signal-transduction molecules, DNA-repair proteins, and chaperone proteins [42-45]. Effects of acetylation of the various groups of nonhistone proteins is shown in Table 2. The opposite effect of deacetylation by interaction with specific HDAC members downregulate the steady state acetylation levels of nonhistone proteins described in Table 2 and attenuate their function. HDAC-mediated deacetylation alters the transcriptional activity of nuclear transcription factors including nuclear factor kappaB (NF-κB) [46-48], p53 [49-53], c-Myb [54, 55], Myo D [56], E2F [57], GATA-1 [58, 59], GATA-2 [60], Fli-1 [61, 62], EKLF [58, 63], Runx 2 [64], Sp1 [65], and Nrf2 [66]. Acetylation of nonhistone chromatin associated HMG (high mobility group) proteins significantly alters their dynamic interactions with the chromatin [67]. This review will discuss the family of HDAC inhibitors which is large and diverse. It includes naturally occuring and synthetic compounds that differ in structure, function, and specificity. HDACIs have demonstrated antitumor activity in clinical trials and had also important therapeutic effects in non-cancer-related diseases such as arthritis, neuromuscular disorders, heart ischemia, cardiac hypertrophy, heart failure and arrhythmias [68], asthma [69, 70], chronic respirating diseases [70], brain disorders such as Rubinstein-Taybi syndrome, Rett syndrome, Friedrich's ataxia, Huntington's disease and multiple sclerosis [71-76], type 1 diabetes [77, 78], hereditary diseases such as human glucose-6-phosphate dehydrogenase deficiency [79], Niemann-Pick type C disease [80, 81], sickle cell anemia [82, 83], malaria [84, 85], and leishmaniasis [86].

DIFFERENT STRUCTURAL GROUPS OF HDAC INHIBITORS

HDACIs can be classified in at least four different groups according to their chemical structure and decreasing potency: hydroxamic acids/ hydroxamates; cyclic peptides, benzamides and short-chain fatty acids (Table 3).

Class III HDACs (sirtuins) are dependent on nicotinamide adenine dinucleotide (NAD) and are therefore inhibited by nicotinamide as derivatives of NAD, dihydrocoumarin, napthopyranone and 2-hydroxynaphaldehydes [84].

Table 2. Effects of acetylation of the various groups of nonhistone proteins

Type of protein HAT	Functional consequence of acetylation	DNA binding transcription factors
DNA binding transcription factors		
NF-κB	p300/CBP, PCAF	Enhanced transcriptional and RelA binding to the NF-κB enhancer
p53	p300/CBP, PCAF	Enhanced DNA binding and protein stabilization.
C-Myb	p300/CBP, GCN5	Enhanced DNA binding (promotes cell proliferation and differentiation).
MyoD	p300/CBP, PCAF	Increased DNA binding (to transactivatemuscle promoters).
E2F	PCAF, p300/CBP	Enhanced DNA binding affinity (to transactivate E2F responsive promotor).
GATA-1	p300/CBP	Enhanced DNA binding activity (stimulation of GATA-1 dependenttranscription).
Fli-1	p300/CBP	Decreased stability of Fli-1 protein and reduced binding to DNA
EKLF	p300/CBP	Enhanced globin gene expression (inhibitory domain modified).
Non-histone chromatin associated proteins		
HMGB1, HMGB2	CBP	Acetylation enhances their ability to bend DNA.
HMGN1, HMGN2	p300	Alters their interaction with chromatin
	p300/PCAF	(weakens their ability to bind to nucleosomal cores).
HMGA	p300/CBP	Enhanceosome disruption (transcription repression).
	PCAF	Enhanceosome assembly (transcription activation).
General transcription factors		
TFIIB	Autoacetylated	Stabilizes interaction between TFIIB and TFIIF and stimulates transcription.
TFIIEb	PCAF, p300/CBP, TAFII50	Unknown
TFIIF	p300, PCAF	Unknown
Viral proteins		
Tat	PCAF	Enhanced transcription (increased CDK9. binding).
	p300/CBP	Enhanced transcription (decreased affinity between Tat and TAR RNA).

Table 3. List of selected HDACI and their properties

Chemical structure class	Compounds	HDAC isoenzyme selectivity	Ref
Hydroxamic acids	Suberoylanilide hydroxamic acid (SAHA; Vorinostat)	Class I, II, IV (HDAC 1-11)	87-90
	Trichostatin A (TSA)	Class I, II, IV (HDAC 1-11)	91-93
	Panobinostat (LBH589)	Class I, II, IV (HDAC 1-11)	94-98
	Belinostat (PXD101)	Class I, II, IV (HDAC 1-11)	99-103
	Quisinostat (JNJ-26481585)	Class I, II, IV (HDAC 1-11)	104-106
	Pracinostat (SB939)	Class I, II, IV (HDAC 1-11)	107-109
	Givinostat (ITF2357)	Class I, II (HDAC 1-10)	110-112
	Abexinostat (PCI-24781)	Class I, II (HDAC 1-10)	113-115
	Resminostat (RAS2410)	Class I, II (HDAC 1-10)	116-118
	Dacinostat (NVP-LAQ 824)	Class I (HDAC 1,2,3, and 8)	119-121
	Suberoylanilide bis-hydroxamic acid	(SBHA)Class I (HDAC 1,3)	122-124
Cyclic peptides	Romidepsin (FK228)	Class Ia (HDAC 1,2)	125-127
	Apicidin	Class I, II (HDAC 1,2,3,4)	128-130
	Trapoxin A	Class I, II (HDAC 1,4)	131,132
Benzamides	Entinostat (MS-275)	Class I (HDAC 1,2,3)	133,134
	Mocetinostat (MGCD0103)	Class I,IV (HDAC 1,2,3,11)	135,136
	Rocilinostat (ACY-1215)	Class IIb (HDAC6)	137-139
	N-acetyl-dinaline (CI-994)	Class I (HDAC 1,2)	140-142
	Chidamide (CS055/HBI-800)	Class I, IIb (HDAC 1,2,3,10)	143
Fatty acids	Sodium butyrate	Class I,IIa,IV (HDAC 1,2, 4,7,5,9,11)	144-146
	Phenyl butyrate	Class I,II (HDAC 1-10)	147-149
	Valproic acid (VPA)	Class I,IIa (HDAC 1,2,4, 7,5,9)	150-154
Mercaptoketone	KD5170	Class I,II (HDAC 1-10)	155-157
Hydroxy-octanediamide derivative	Tubacin (tubulin acetylation inducer)	specific HDAC 6 inhibitor	158-160
Thiazoline-oxazole largazole analogs		Class I	161-163

Trichostatin A (TSA) was the first natural hydroxamate found as HDACs inhibitor [164]. Vorinostat (suberoylanilide hydroxamic acid, Zolinza), which is structurally similar to TSA, was the first HDACI approved on October 6, 2006 by US Food and Drug Administration (FDA) for the treatment of relapsed and refractory cutaneous T-cell lymphoma (CTCL) [165]. The hydroxamates include also panobinostat (LBH589), belinostat (PXD101), quisinostat (JNJ-26481585), pracinostat (SB939), givinostat (ITF2357), abexinostat (PCI-24781), resminostat (RAS2410), dacinostat (NVP-LAQ 824), and suberoylanilide bis-hydroxamic acid (SBHA) (Table 3). Resminostat was approved on Septeber 6, 2011 for patients with Hodgkinś lymphoma [166]. The cyclic peptides include romidepsin (FK228, Istodax), apicidin and tropoxin A.

Based on two large Phase II studies, the US FDA approved intravenous romidepsin for patients with relapsed and refractory CTCL on November 6, 2009 [167]. The majority of HDACIs of these two groups are very potent with activity within the nanomolar range. Other HDACIs from these two groups (belinostat, panobiostat, resminostat, quisinostat) are effective in micromolar range similarly as the further group (benzamides). Benzamides include entinostat (MS-275), mocetinostat (MGCD0103), rocilinostat (ACY-1215), N-acetyl-dinaline (CI-994), and chidamide (CS055/HBI-800). Fatty acids (sodium butyrate, phenyl butyrate, and valproic acid) are efficient within the milimolar range. The hydroxamates are generally nonspecific HDACIs affecting all classes of HDACs. Other groups are more specific HDACIs (Table 3).

MECHANISMS OF HDAC INHIBITORS ACTION

Lysine sites on proteins acetylation plays an important role in major cellular functions including DNA damage repair, cell cycle progression, immune pathways, cell migration and adhesion, and angiogenesis [168]. The response to DNA damage is regulated by HDACIs by coordinating DNA damage checkpoints and double-strand DNA break processing with autophagy [169-171]. HDACIs increase histone acetylation, which subsequently downregulates transcription factors involved in promoting cell cycle progression and upregulates proteins that block cell cycle progression [172, 173]. HDACIs cause the upregulation of the cyclin-dependent kinase inhibitor $p21^{WAF1/CIP1}$ and subsequently block the cell cycle in G1 phase in malignant cells. HDACIs downregulate cyclins and dephosphorylate retinoblastoma protein. HDACIs are potent inducers of apoptosis and pro- and anti-apoptotic factors are their modulated targets [174, 175]. HDACIs downregulate prosurvival proteins such as Bcl-2 and upregulate pro-apoptotic proteins such as Bax, Bak and Bim. The therapeutic effects of HDACIs may be explained by the dual role of autophagy in disease progress [173, 176-178]. HDACIs block angiogenesis by downregulating angiogenesis stimulating factor HIF-1α (hypoxia inducible factor 1α) and VEGF (vascular endothelial growth factor) [179, 180]. Accumulation of reactive oxygen species (ROS) in malignant cells is the further important mechanism of HDACIs-mediated cell death [181, 182]. Chaperone function is critical in the stability of numerous proteins, including some important oncoproteins and tumor suppressors. HDACIs inactivate and interfere the binding of HSP90 (heat shock protein 90) to these client proteins, leading to their instability and degradation [183-185]. HDAC6 is a regulatory component of aggresome and targeted inhibition of HDAC6 causes autophagic cell death in tumor cells [186, 187]. All these HDACI-activated antitumor pathways are in detail described in several reviews [19, 173, 188].

HDAC Inhibitors in Cancer Therapy

Drug discovery has always been a complex process including many steps from target validation to clinical development. As upper described, vorinostat, romidepsin, and resminostat were approved by US FDA for cancer therapy. Tens of structurally disparate HDACIs are under different stages of clinical trials [21, 22, 189]. Panobinostat (LBH589) is in phase III clinical trial and shows clinical effects in CTCL patients with a rapid change of the expression of genes involved in apoptosis, immune regulation and angiogenesis [94, 190]. LBH589 is also in phase II clinical trials in further hematological diseases, such as Hodgkin lymphoma (HL), myeloma, myeloid malignancies, and Waldenstrom's macroglobulinemia (WM) [21, 94]. The results of Phase II trials prove that oral panobinostat is deliverable with dosing regimens of three times per week, either weekly or biweekly. The major hematologic side-effect of myelosuppression, in particular thrombocytopenia, is transient and manageable, as are the non-hematologic side-effects. Encouraging responses are observed in HL, CTCL, myelofibrosis and WM. The safety and efficacy results from studies of combination therapy with azacitidine in acute myeloid leukemia and myelodysplastic syndromes suggest that this agent may find a place in the management of a range of hematologic cancers [94]. LBH589 did not dramatically change the outcome of leukemia, when used as single agent [21]. However, it has to be considered that nearly all the completed trials have been conducted on refractory-relapsed heavily treated patients, where adjunctive molecular changes and mechanisms of drug resistance might have occured.

HDACIs used in combination therapy are also studied in many clinical trials [21, 23, 172]. Combining HDACIs and topoisomerase inhibitors, radiotherapy, DNA methyltransferase inhibitors, histone methylation inhibitors, hormonal therapy, tyrosine kinase inhibitors, multikinase inhibitor, mTOR inhibitor, and proteasome inhibitors are studied [23, 172, 191-197].

In recent years many kinds of HDACI biomarkers have been used to predict response of these drugs [166]. Histone acetylation, induction of p21 and Hsp90, HDAC enzyme activity, gene signatures, HDAC enzyme expression, the protein HR23B, tolerances to oxidative stress, and level of phosphocholine are used as predictive biomarkers for HDACI-based therapy [166].

Adverse Events of HDAC Inhibitors

Nausea, vomiting, and anorexia were the most common higher grade adverse events observed with the use of HDACIs [198]. Fatigue is a common side effect seen with all HDACIs, and the symptom rapidly resolves upon drug discontinuation. From hematologic side effects, thrombocytopenia, neutropenia and anemia were observed following HDACIs administration. Arrythmias have been also reported in patients treated with HDACIs. Liver toxicities and neurological events were also noted. These toxicities were observed in single agent studies.

Conclusion and Perspective

HDACs are critical modulators of disorders such as cancer and inflammatory diseases. The development of HDACIs as anti-tumor drugs is very important for cancer therapeutics. While the underlying mechanisms are under intensive study, there are several questions that need to be answered regarding to the clinical use of HDACIs. It is necessary to explain why HDACIs specifically target tumor cells, while normal non-malignant cells remained largely unaltered? For example, the association between HDACI activity and induction of DNA damage has long been recognized [199]. HDACIs are able to perturb DNA damage response [200]. The specificity of HDACIs in cancer therapy should also be questioned. Clinical responses diversify between different HDACIs which target the same HDACs. To address this problem, more isoform-specific HDACIs may be needed. The mechanistic base of the resistance to HDACIs needs also further study. Clinical trials for combination therapies using HDACIs together with other drugs will provide more clinical experience and new strategies in fighting cancer.

ACKNOWLEDGMENTS

This work was supported by research project (Ministry of Health, Czech Republic) for conceptual development of research organization (00023736; Institute of Hematology and Blood Transfusion, Prague).

REFERENCES

[1] Allfrey VG, Faulkner R, Mirsky AE. Acetylation and methylation of histones and their possible role in the regulation of RNA synthesis. *Proc. Natl. Acad. Sci. USA* 1964, 51, 786-794.

[2] Bannister Aj, Kouzarides T. Regulation of chromatin by histone modifications. *Cell Res.* 2011, 21, 381-395.

[3] Kiermaier A, Eilers M. Transcriptional control: Calling in histone deacetylase. *Curr. Biol.* 1997, 7, R505-R507.

[4] Hassig CA, Schreiber SL. Nuclear histone acetylases and deacetylases and transcriptional regulation: HATs off to HDACs. *Curr. Opin. Chem. Biol.* 1997, 1, 300-308.

[5] Kuo MH, Allis CD. Role of histone acetyltransferases and deacetylases in gene regulation. *BioEssays* 1998, 20, 615-626.

[6] Luo RX, Dean DC. Chromatin remodeling and transcriptional regulation. *J. Natl. Cancer Inst.* 1999, 91, 1288-1294.

[7] Johnson CA, Turner BM. Histone deacetylases: complex transducers of nuclear signals. *Semin. Cell Dev. Biol.* 1999, 10, 179-188.

[8] Cress WD, Seto E. Histone deacetylases, transcriptional control, and cancer. *J. Cell. Physiol.* 2000, 184, 1-16.

[9] Wade PA. Transcriptional control regulatory checkpoints by histone deacetylases: molecular connections between cancer and chromatin. *Hum. Mol. Genet.* 2001, 10, 693-698.

[10] Gray SG, Ekström TJ. The human histone deacetylase family. *Exp. Cell Res.* 2001, 262, 75-83.

[11] Khochbin S, Kao HY. Histone deacetylase complexes: functional entities or molecular reservoirs. *FEBS Lett.* 2001, 494, 141-144.

[12] Walkinshaw DR, Tahmasebi S, Bertos NR, Yang XJ. Histone deacetylases as transducers and targets of nuclear signaling. *J. Cell. Biochem.* 2008, 104, 1541-1552.

[13] Marks PA, Richon VM, Breslow R, Rifkind RA. Histone deacetylase inhibitors as new cancer drugs. *Curr. Opin. Oncol.* 2001, 13, 477-483.

[14] Tong JK. Dissecting histone deacetylase function. *Chem. Biol.* 2002, 9, 668-670.

[15] Sengupta N, Seto E. Regulation of histone deacetylase activities. *J. Cell. Biochem.* 2004, 93, 56-67.

[16] Monneret C. Histone deacetylase inhibitors. *Eur. J. Med. Chem.* 2005, 40, 1-13.

[17] Marks PA, Jiang X. Histone deacetylase inhibitors in programmed cell death and cancer therapy. *Cell Cycle* 2005,4, 549-551.

[18] Kouraklis G, Misiakos EP, Theocharis S. Histone deacetylase inhibitors as a potential therapeutic agent for human cancer treatment. *Targ. Oncol.* 2006, 1, 34-41.

[19] Marks PA, Xu WS. Histone deacetylase inhibitors: potential in cancer therapy. *J. Cell. Biochem.* 2009, 107, 600-608.

[20] Lane AA, Chabner BA. Histone deacetylase inhibitors in cancer therapy. *J. Clin. Oncol.* 2009, 27, 5459-5468.

[21] Tambaro FP, Dell'Aversana C, Carafa V, Nebbioso A, Radic B, Ferrara F, Altucci L. Histone deacetylase inhibitors: clinical implications for hematological malignancies. *Clin Epigenet.* 2010, 1, 25-44.

[22] Kim HJ, Bae SC. Histone deacetylase inhibitors: molecular mechanisms of action and clinical trials as anti-cancer drugs. *Am. J. Transl. Res.* 2011, 3, 166-179.

[23] Thurn KT, Thomas S, Moore A, Munster PN. Rational therapeutic combinations with histone deacetylase inhibitors for the treatment of cancer. *Future Oncol.* 2011, 7, 263-283.

[24] Kroesen M, Gielen PR, Brok IC, Armandari I, Hoogerbrugge PM, Adema GJ. HDAC inhibitors and immunotherapy; a double edged sword? *Oncotarget* 2014, 5, 6558-6572.

[25] Falkenberg KJ, Johnstone RW. Histone deacetylases and their inhibitors in cancer, neurological diseases and immune disorders. *Nat. Rev. Drug Discov.* 2014, 13, 673-691.

[26] West AC, Johnstone RW. New and emerging HDAC inhibitors in cancer treatment. *J. Clin. Invest.* 2014, 124, 30-39.

[27] Li Z, Zhu WG. Targeting histone deacetylases for cancer therapy: from molecular mechanisms to clinical implications. *Int. J. Biol. Sci.* 2014, 10, 757-770.

[28] Zhang J, Zhong Q. Histone deacetylase inhibitors and cell death. *Cell. Mol. Life Sci.* 2014, 71, 3885-3901.

[29] Kornberg RD. Chromatin structure: a repeating unit of histones and DNA. *Science* 1974, 184, 868-871.

[30] Kornberg RD. Structure of chromatin. *Annu. Rev. Biochem.* 1977, 46, 931-954.

[31] de Ruijter AJ, van Gennip AH, Caron HN, Kemp S, van Kuilenburg AB. Histone deacetylases (HDACs): characterization of the classical HDAC family. *Biochem. J.* 2003, 370, 737-749.

[32] Gregoretti IV, Lee YM, Goodson HV. Molecular evolution of the histone deacetylase family: functional implications of phylogenetic analysis. *J. Mol. Biol.* 2004, 338, 17-31.

[33] Tanner KG, Landry J, Sternglanz R, Denu JM. Silent information regulator 2 family of NAD-dependent histone/protein deacetylases generates a unique product, 1-O-acetyl-ADP-ribose. *Proc. Natl. Acad. Sci. U S A.* 2000, 97, 14178–14182.

[34] Vaquero A. The conserved role of sirtuins in chromatin regulation. *Int. J. Dev. Biol.* 2009, 53, 303-322.

[35] Sanders BD, Jackson B, Marmorstein R. Structural basis for sirtuin function: what we know and what we don't. *Biochim. Biophys. Acta* 2010, 1804, 1604-1616.

[36] Martinez-Redondo P, Vaquero A. The diversity of histone versus nonhistone sirtuin substrates. *Genes Cancer* 2013, 47, 148-163.

[37] Roth M, Wang Z, Chen WY. Sirtuins in hematological aging and malignancy. *Crit. Rev. Oncog.* 2013, 18, 531-547.

[38] Yang XJ, Seto E. The Rpd3/Hda1 family of lysine deacetylases: from bacteria and yeast to mice and men. *Nat. Rev. Mol. Cell Biol.* 2008, 9, 206–218.

[39] Martin M, Kettmann R, Dequiedt F. Class IIa histone deacetylases: regulating the regulators. *Oncogene* 2007, 26, 5450–5467.

[40] Marks PA. Histone deacetylase inhibitors: a chemical genetics approach to understanding cellular functions. *Biochim. Biophys. Acta.* 2010, 1799, 717–725.

[41] Ocker M. Deacetylase inhibitors – focus on non-histone targets and effects. *World J. Biol. Chem.* 2010,1, 55–61.

[42] Glozak MA, Sengupta N, Zhang X, Seto E. Acetylation and deacetylation of non-histone proteins. *Gene* 2005, 363, 15–23.

[43] Das C, Kundu TK. Transcriptional regulation by the acetylation of nonhistone proteins in humans-a new target for therapeutics. *IUBMB Life* 2005, 57, 137-148.

[44] Spange S, Wagner T, Heinzel T, Krämer OH. Acetylation of non-histone proteins modulates cellular signalling at multiple levels. *Int. J. Biochem. Cell Biol.* 2009, 41, 185-198.

[45] Yao YL, Yang WM. Beyond histone and deacetylase: an overview of cytoplasmic histone deacetylases and their nonhistone substrates. *J. Biomed. Biotechnol.* 2011, Article ID 146493, 15 pages.

[46] Chen LF, Mu Y, Greene WC. Acetylation of RelA at discrete sites regulates distinct nuclear functions of NF-κB. *EMBO J.* 2002, 21, 6539-6548.

[47] Kiernan R, Bres V, Ng RW, Coudart MP, El MS, Sardet C, Jin DY, Emiliani S, Benkirane M. Post-activation turn-off of NF-κB-dependent transcription is regulated by acetylation of p65. *J. Biol. Chem.* 2003, 278, 2758-2766.

[48] Huang B, Yang XD, Lamb A, Chen LF. Posttranslational modifications of NF-κB: another layer of regulation for NF-κB signaling pathway. *Cell Signal.* 2010, 22, 1282-1290.

[49] Gu W, Roeder RG. Activation of p53 sequence-specific DNA binding by acetylation of the p53 C-terminal domain. *Cell* 1997, 90, 595-606.

[50] Luo J, Su F, Chen D, Shiloh A, Gu W. Deacetylation of p53 modulates its effect on cell growth and apoptosis. *Nature* 2000, 408, 377-381.

[51] Brooks CL, Gu W. Ubiquitination, phosphorylation and acetylation: the molecular basis for p53 regulation. *Curr. Opin. Cell Biol.* 2003, 15, 164-171.

[52] Harms KL, Chen X. Histone deacetylase 2 modulates p53 transcriptional activities through regulation of p53-DNA binding activity. *Cancer Res.* 2007, 67, 3145-3152.

[53] Contreras AU, Mebratu Y, Delgado M, Montamo G, Hu CA, Ryter SW, Choi AM, Lin Y, Xiang J, Chaud H, Tesfaigzi Y. *J. Cell Biol.* 2013, 201, 427-437.

[54] Tomita A, Towatari M, Tsuzuki S, Hayakawa F, Kosugi H, Tamai K, Miyazaki T, Kinoshita T, Saito H. c-Myb acetylation at the carboxy-terminal conserved domain by transcriptional co-activator p300. *Oncogene* 2000, 19, 444-451.

[55] Tsai SC, Seto E. Increased affinity of c-Myb for CREB-binding protein (CBP) after CBP-induced acetylation. *J. Biol. Chem.* 2001, 276, 3674-3682.

[56] Poleskaya A, Duquat A, Naguibueva I, Weise C, Vervisch A, Bengal E, Hucho F, Robin P, Harel-Bellan A. A CREB-binding protein/p300 activates MyoD by acetylation. *J. Biol. Chem.* 2000, 275, 34359-34364.

[57] Botillier AL, Trinh E, Loeffler JP. Selective E2F-dependent gene transcription is controlled by histone deacetylase activity during neuronal apoptosis. *J. Neurochem.* 2003, 84, 814-828.

[58] Huo X, Zhang J. Important roles of reversible acetylation in the function of hematopoietic transcription factors. *J. Cell. Mol. Med.* 2005, 9, 103-112.

[59] Boyes J, Byfield P, Nakatani Y, Ogryzko V. Regulation of activity of the transcription factor GATA-1 by acetylation. *Nature* 1998, 396, 594-598.

[60] Hayakawa F, Towatari M, Ozawa Y, Tomita A, Privalsky ML, Saito H. Functional regulation of GATA-2 by acetylation. *J. Leukoc. Biol.* 2004, 75, 529-540.

[61] Asano Y, Czuwara J, Trojanowska M. Transforming growth factor-β regulates DNA binding activity of transcription factor Fli1 by p300/CREB-binding protein-associated factor-dependent acetylation. *J. Biol. Chem.* 2007, 282, 3472-3483.

[62] Asano Y, Trojanowska M. Fli1 represses transcription of the human α2 (I) collagen gene by recruitment HDAC1/p300 complex. *PLOS One* 2013, 8, e74930.

[63] Zhang W, Bieker JJ. Acetylation and modulation of erythroid Krüppel-like factor (EKLF) activity by interaction with acetyltransferases. *Proc. Natl. Acad. Sci. USA* 1998, 95, 9855-9860.

[64] Jeon EJ, Lee KY, Choi NS, Lee MH, Kim HN, Jin YH, Ryoo HM, Choi JY, Yoshida M, Nishino N, Oh BC, Lee KS, Lee YH, Bae SC. Bone morphogenetic protein-2 stimulates Runx 2 acetylation. *J. Biol. Chem.* 2006, 281, 16502-16511.

[65] Hung JJ, Wang YT, Chang WC. Sp1 deacetylation induces by phorbol ester recruits p300 to activate 12(S)-lipoxygenase gene transcription. *Mol. Cell Biol.* 2006, 26, 1770-1785.

[66] Kawai Y, Garduno L, Theodore M, Yang J, Arinze IJ. Acetylation-deacetylation of the transcription factor Nrf 2 (nuclear factor erythroid 2-related factor 2) regulates its transcriptional activity and nucleocytoplasmic localization. *J. Biol. Chem.* 2011, 286, 7629-7640.

[67] Bergel M, Herrera JE, Thatcher BJ, Prymakowska-Bosck M, Vassilev A, Nakatani Y, Martin B, Bustin M. Acetylation of novel sites in the nucleosomal binding domain of chromosomal protein HMG-14 by p300 alters its interaction with nucleosomes. *J. Biol. Chem.* 2000, 275, 11514-11520.

[68] Colussi C, Illi B, Rosati J, Spallotta F, Farsetti A, Grasselli A, Mai A, Capogrossi MC, Gaetano C. Histone deacetylase inhibitors: keeping momentum for neuromuscular and cardiovascular diseases treatment. *Pharmacol. Res.* 2010, 62, 3-10.

[69] Royce SG, Ververis K, Karagiannis TC. Histone deacetylase inhibitors: can we considerpotent anti-neoplastic agents for the treatment of asthma? *Ann. Clin. Lab. Sci.* 2012, 42, 338-345.

[70] Royce SG, Karagiannis TC. Histone deacetylases and their inhibitors: new implications for asthma and chronic respiratory conditions. *Curr. Opin. Allergy Clin. Immunol.* 2014, 14, 44-48.

[71] Kazantsev AG, Thompson LM. Therapeutic application of histone deacetylase inhibitors for central nervous system disorders. *Nat. Rev. Drug Discov.* 2008, 7, 854-868.

[72] Soragni E, Xu C, Cooper A, Plasterer HL, Rusche JR, Gottaseld JM. Evaluation of histone deacetylase inhibitors as therapeutics for neurodegenerative diseases. *Methods Mol. Biol.* 2011, 793, 495-508.

[73] Abdel-Magid AF. Histone deacetylase 4 (HDAC 4) inhibitors: a promising treatment for Huntington disease, *ACS Med. Chem. Lett.* 2013, 4, 692-693.

[74] Harrison IF, Dexter DT. Epigenetic targeting of histone deacetylase: therapeutic potential in Parkinson's disease? *Pharmacol. Ther.* 2013, 140, 34-52.

[75] Thomas EA. Involvement of HDAC1 and HDAC3 in the pathology of polyglutamine disorders: therapeutic implications for selective HDAC1/HDAC3 inhibitors. *Pharmaceuticals* (Basel) 2014, 7, 634-661.

[76] Cacabelos R, Torrellas C. Epigenetic drug discovery for Alzheimer's disease. *Expert Opin. Drug Discov.* 2014, 9, 1059-1086.

[77] Jayaraman S. Novel methods of type 1 diabetes treatment. *Discov. Med.* 2014, 17, 347-355.

[78] Christensen DP, Gysemans C, Lundh M, Dahllöf MS, Noesgaard D, Schmidt SF, Mandrup S, Birkbak N, Workman CT, Piemonti L, Blaabjerg L, Monzani V, Fossati G, Mascagni P, Paraskevas S, Aikin RA, Billestrup N, Grunnet LG, Dinarello CA, Mathieu C, Mandrup-Poulsen T. Lysine deacetylase inhibition prevents diabetes by chromatin-independent immunoregulation and β-cell protection. *Proc. Natl. Acad. Sci. USA* 2014, 111, 1055-1059.

[79] Makarona K, Caputo VS, Costa JR, Lin B, O'Connor D, Iksander D, Roper D, Robertson L, Bhatnagar N, Terpos E, Georgiou E, Papaivannon M, Layton DM, Luzzato L, Roberts I, Karadimitros A. Transcriptional and epigenetic basis for restoration of G6PD enzymatic activity in human G6PD-deficient cells. *Blood* 2014, 124, 131-141.

[80] Helquist P, Maxfield FR, Wiech NL, Wiest O. Treatment of Niemann-Pick type C disease by histone deacetylase inhibitors. *Neurotherapeutics* 2013, 10, 688-697.

[81] Maceyka M, Milstein S, Spiegel S. The potential of histone deacetylase inhibitors in Niemann-Pick type C disease. *FEBS J.* 2013, 280, 6367-6372.

[82] Eridani S, Mosca A. Fetal hemoglobin reactivation and cell engineering in the treatment of sickle cell anemia. *J. Blood Med.* 2011, 2, 23-30.

[83] Okam MM, Ebert BL. Novel approaches to the treatment of sickle cell disease: the potential of histone deacetylase inhibitors. *Expert Rev. Hematol.* 2012, 5, 303-311.

[84] Andrews KT, Tran TN, Wheatley NC, Fairlie DP. Targeting histone deacetylase inhibitors for anti-malarial therapy. *Curr. Top. Med. Chem.* 2009, 9, 292-308.

[85] Sumanadasa SD[1], Goodman CD, Lucke AJ, Skinner-Adams T, Sahama I, Haque A, Do TA, McFadden GI, Fairlie DP, Andrews KT. Antimalarial activity of the anticancer histone deacetylase inhibitor SB939. *Antimicrob. Agents Chemother.* 2012, 56, 3849-3856.

[86] Sodji Q, Patil V, Jain S, Kornacki JR, Mrksich M, Tekwani BL, Oyelere AK. The antileishmanial activity of isoforms 6- and 8-selective histone deacetylase inhibitors. *Bioorg. Med. Chem. Lett.* 2014, 24, 4826-4830.

[87] Kelly WK, Marks PA. Drug insight: Histone deacetylase inhibitors--development of the new targeted anticancer agent suberoylanilide hydroxamic acid. *Nat. Clin. Pract. Oncol.* 2005, 2, 150-157.

[88] Hrzenjak A, Moinfar F, Kremser ML, Strohmeier B, Betru E, Zatloukal K, Denk H. Histone deacetylase inhibitor vorinostat suppresses the growth of uterine sarcomas in vitro and in vivo. *Mol. Cancer* 2010, 9, 49.

[89] Brodská B, Holoubek A, Otevřelová P, Kuželová K. Combined treatment with low concentrations of decitabine and SAHA casuses cell death in leukemic cell lines but not in normal peripheral blood lymphocytes. *Biomed. Res. Int.* 2013, 2013, 659254.

[90] Iwamoto M, Friedman EJ, Sandhu P, Agrawal NG, Rubin EH, Wagner JA. Clinical pharmacology profile of vorinostat, a histone deacetylase inhibitor. *Cancer Chemother. Pharmacol.* 2013, 72, 493-508.

[91] Kim YB, Yoshida M, Horinouchi S. Selective induction of cyclin-dependent kinase inhibitors and their roles in cell cycle arrest caused by trichostatin A, an inhibitor of histone deacetylase. *Ann. NY Acad. Sci.* 1999, 886, 200-203.

[92] Vanhaecke T, Papeleu P, Elaut G, Rogiers V. Trichostatin A – like hydroxamate histone deacetylase inhibitors as therapeutic agents: toxicological point of view. *Curr. Med. Chem.* 2004, 11, 1129-1143.

[93] Peiffer L, Poll-Wolbeck SJ, Flamme H, Gehrke I, Hallek M, Kreuzer KA. Trichostatin A effectively induces apoptosis in chronic lymphocytic leukemia cells via inhibition of Wnt signaling and histone deacetylation. *J. Cancer Res. Clin. Oncol.* 2014, 140, 1283-1293.

[94] Khot A, Dickinson M, Prince HM. Panobinostat in lymphoid and myeloid malignancies. *Expert Opin. Investig. Drugs* 2013, 22, 1211-1223.

[95] Anne M, Sammartino D, Barginear MF, Budman D. Profile of panobinostat and its potential for treatment in solid tumors: an update. *OncoTargets Therapy* 2013, 6, 1613-1624.

[96] Fortunati N, Marano F, Bandino A, Frairia R, Catalano MG, Boccuzzi G. The pan-histone deacetylase inhibitor LBH 589 (panobinostat) alters the invasive breast cancer cell phenotype. *Int. J. Oncol.* 2014, 44, 700-708.

[97] Li X, Zhang J, Xie Y, Jiang Y, Yingjie Z, Xu W. Progress of HDAC inhibitor panobinostat in the treatment of cancer. *Curr. Drug Targets* 2014, 15, 622-634.

[98] Rajkumar SV. Panobinostat for the treatment of multiple myeloma. *Lancet Oncol.* 2014, 15, 1178-1179.

[99] Gimsing P, Hansen M, Knudsen LM, Knoblauch P, Christensen IJ, Ooi CE, Buhl-Jensen P. A phase I clinical trial of the histone deacetylase

inhibitor belinostat in patients with advanced hematological neoplasia. *Eur. J. Haematol.* 2008, 81, 170-176.

[100] Gimsing P. Belinostat: a new broad acting antineoplastic histone deacetylase inhibitor. *Expert Opin. Investig. Drugs* 2009, 18, 501-508.

[101] Steele NL, Plumb JA, Vidal L, Tjørnclund J, Knoblauch P, Buhl-Jensen P, Molife R, Brown R, de Bono JS, Evans TR. Pharmacokinetic and pharmacodynamic properties of an oral formulation of the histone deacetylase inhibitor Belinostat (PXD101). *Cancer Chemother. Pharmacol.* 2011, 67, 1273-1279.

[102] Poole RM. Belinostat: first global approval. *Drugs* 2014, 74, 1543-1554.

[103] McDermott J, Jimeno A. Belinostat for the treatment of peripheral T-cell lymphomas. *Drugs Today (Barc).* 2014, 50, 337-345.

[104] Stühmer T, Arts J, Chatterjee M, Borawski J, Wolff A, King P, Einsele H, Leo E, Bargou RC. Preclinical anti-myeloma activity of the novel HDAC-inhibitor JNJ-26481585. *Br. J. Haematol.* 2010, 149, 529-536.

[105] Arts J, King P, Mariën A, Floren W, Beliën A, Janssen L, Pilatte I, Roux B, Decrane L, Gilissen R, Hickson I, Vreys V, Cox, Bol K, Talloen W, Goris I, Andries L, Du Jardin M, Janicot M, Page, van Emelen K, Angibaud P. JNJ-26481585, a novel "second-generation" oral histone deacetylase inhibitor, shows broad-spectrum preclinical antitumoral activity. *Clin. Cancer Res.* 2009, 15, 6841-6851.

[106] Tong WG, Wei Y, Stevenson W, Kuang SQ, Fang Z, Zhang M, Arts J, Garcia-Manero G. Preclinical antileukemia activity of JNJ-26481585, a potent second-generation histone deacetylase inhibitor. *Leuk. Res.* 2010, 34, 221-228.

[107] Novotny-Diermayr V, Sangthongpitag K, Hu CY, Wu X, Sausgruber N, Yeo P, Greicius G, Pettersson S, Liang AL, Loh YK, Bonday Z, Goh KC, Hentze H, Hart S, Wang H, Ethirajulu K, Wood JM. SB939, a novel potent and orally active histone deacetylase inhibitor with high tumor exposure and efficacy in mouse models of colorectal cancer. *Mol. Cancer Ther.* 2010, 9, 642-652.

[108] Razak AR, Hotte SJ, Siu LL, Chen EX, Hirte HW, Powers J, Walsh W, Stayner LA, Laughlin A, Novotny-Diermayr V, Zhu J, Eisenhauer EA. Phase I clinical, pharmacokinetic and pharmacodynamic study of SB939, an oral histone deacetylase (HDAC) inhibitor, in patients with advanced solid tumours. *Br. J. Cancer* 2011, 104, 756-762.

[109] Yong WP, Goh BC, Soo RA, Toh HC, Ethirajulu K, Wood J, Novotny-Diermayr V, Lee SC, Yeo WL, Chan D, Lim D, Seah E, Lim R, Zhu J. Phase I and pharmacodynamic study of an orally administered novel

inhibitor of histone deacetylases, SB939, in patients with refractory solid malignancies. *Ann. Oncol.* 2011, 22, 2516-2522.

[110] Golay J, Cuppini L, Leoni F, Micó C, Barbui V, Domenghini M, Lombardi L, Neri A, Barbui AM, Salvi A, Pozzi P, Porro G, Pagani P, Fossati G, Mascagni G, Introna M, Rambaldi A. The histone deacetylase inhibitor ITF2357 has anti-leukemic aktivity in vitro and in vivo and inhibits IL-6 and VEGF production by stromal cells. *Leukemia* 2007, 21, 1892-1900.

[111] Barbetti V, Gozzini A, Rovida E, Morandi A, Spinelli E, Fossati G, Mascagni P, Lübbert M, Dello Sharba P, Santini V. Selective anti-leukemic aktivity of low dose histone deacetylase inhibitor ITF2357 on AML1/ETO – positive cells. *Oncogene* 2008, 27, 1767-1778.

[112] Amaru Calzada A, Todverti K, Donadoni L, Pellicioli A, Tuana G, Gatta R, Neri A, Finazzi G, Mantovani R, Rambaldi A, Introna M, Lombardi L, Golay J, AGIM investigators. The HDAC inhibitor Givinostat modulates the hematopoietic transcription factors NFE2 and c-MYB in JAK2 (V617F) myeloproliferative neoplasm cells.

[113] Rivera-Del Valle N, Gao S, Miller CP, Fulbright J, Gonzales C, Sirisawad M, Steggerda S, Wheler J, Balasubramanian S, Chandra J. PCI-24781, a Novel Hydroxamic Acid HDAC Inhibitor, Exerts Cytotoxicity and Histone Alterations via Caspase-8 and FADD in Leukemia Cells. *Int. J. Cell. Biol.* 2010, 2010, 207420.

[114] Yang C, Choy E, Hornicek FJ, Wood KB, Schwab JH, Liu X, Mankin H, Duan Z. Histone deacetylase inhibitor PCI-24781 enhances chemotherapy-induced apoptosis in multidrug-resistant sarcoma cell lines. *Anticancer Res.* 2011, 31, 1115-1123.

[115] Fouliard S, Robert R, Jacquet-Bescond A, du Rieu QC, Balasubramanian S, Loury D, Loriot Y, Hollebecque A, Kloos I, Soria JC, Chenel M, Depil S. Pharmacokinetic/pharmacodynamic modelling-based optimisation of administration schedule for the histone deacetylase inhibitor abexinostat (S78454/PCI-24781) in phase I. *Eur. J. Cancer* 2013, 49, 2791-2797.

[116] Mandl-Weber S, Meinel FG, Jankowsky R, Oduncu F, Schmidmaier R, Baumann P. The novel inhibitor of histone deacetylase resminostat (RAS2410) inhibits proliferation and induces apoptosis in multiple myeloma (MM) cells. *Br. J. Haematol.* 2010, 149, 518-528.

[117] Brunetto AT, Ang JE, Lal R, Olmos D, Molife LR, Kristeleit R, Parker A, Casamayor I, Olaleye M, Mais A, Hauns B, Strobel V, Hentsch B, de Bono JS. *Clin. Cancer Res.* 2013, 19, 5494-5504.

[118] Rajak H, Singh A, Raghuwanshi K, Kumar R, Dewangan PK, Veerasamy R, Sharma PC, Dixit A, Mishra P. A structural insight into hydroxamic acid based histone deacetylase inhibitors for the presence of anticancer activity. *Curr. Med. Chem.* 2014, 21, 2642-2664.

[119] Remiszewski SW. The discovery of NVP-LAQ824: from concept to clinic. *Curr. Med. Chem.* 2003, 10, 2393-2402.

[120] Rosato RR, Almenara JA, Maggio SC, Coe S, Atadja P, Dent P, Grant S. Role of histone deacetylase inhibitor-induced reactive oxygen species and DNA damage in LAQ-824/fludarabine antileukemic interactions. *Mol. Cancer Ther.* 2008, 7, 3285-3297.

[121] de Bono JS, Kristeleit R, Tolcher A, Fong P, Pacey S, Karavasilis V, Mita M, Shaw H, Workman P, Kaye S, Rowinsky EK, Aherne W, Atadja P, Scott JW, Patnaik A. Phase I pharmacokinetic and pharmacodynamic study of LAQ824, a hydroxamate histone deacetylase inhibitor with a heat shock protein-90 inhibitory profile, in patients with advanced solid tumors. *Clin. Cancer Res.* 2008, 14, 6663-6673.

[122] Zhang XD, Gillespie SK, Borrow JM, Hersey P. The histone deacetylase inhibitor suberic bishydroxamate: a potential sensitizer of melanoma to TNF-related apoptosis-inducing ligand (TRAIL) induced apoptosis. *Biochem. Pharmacol.* 2003, 66, 1537-1545.

[123] Zhang XD, Gillespie SK, Borrow JM, Hersey P. The histone deacetylase inhibitor suberic bishydroxamate regulates the expression of multiple apoptotic mediators and induces mitochondria-dependent apoptosis of melanoma cells. *Mol. Cancer Ther.* 2004, 3, 425-435.

[124] You BR, Park WH. Suberoyl bishydroxamic acid inhibits the growth of A549 lung cancer cells via caspase-dependent apoptosis. *Mol. Cell. Biochem.* 2010, 344, 203-210.

[125] Furumai R, Matsuyama A, Kobashi N, Lee KH, Nishiyama M, Nakajima H, Tanaka A, Komatsu Y, Nishino N, Yoshida M, Horinouchi S. FK228 (depsipeptide) as a natural prodrug that inhibits class I histone deacetylases. *Cancer Res.* 2002, 62, 4916-4921.

[126] Newbold A, Lindemann RK, Cluse LA, Whitecross KF, Dear AE, Johnstone RW. Characterisation of the novel apoptotic and therapeutic activities of the histone deacetylase inhibitor romidepsin. *Mol. Cancer Ther.* 2008, 7, 1066-1079.

[127] Bertino EM, Otterson GA. Romidepsin: a novel histone deacetylase inhibitor for cancer. *Expert Opin. Investig. Drugs* 2011, 20, 1151-1158.

[128] Ahn MY, Lee J, Na YJ, Choi WS, Lee BM, Kang KW, Kim HS. Mechanism of apicidin-induced cell cycle arrest and apoptosis in

Ishikawa human endometrial cancer cells. *Chem. Biol. Interact.* 2009, 179, 169-177.

[129] Chang J, Varghese DS, Gillam MC, Peyton M, Modi B, Schiltz RL, Girard L, Martinez ED. Differential response of cancer cells to HDAC inhibitors trichostatin A and depsipeptide. *Br. J. Cancer* 2012, 106, 116-125.

[130] Ahn MY, Kang DO, Na YJ, Yoon S, Choi WS, Kang KW, Chung HY, Jung JH, Min do S, Kim HS. Histone deacetylase inhibitor, apicidin, inhibits human ovarian cancer cell migration via class II histone deacetylase 4 silencing. *Cancer Lett.* 2012, 325, 189-199.

[131] Kijima M, Yoshida M, Sugita K, Horinouchi S, Beppu T. Trapoxin, an antitumor cyclic tetrapeptide, is an irreversible inhibitor of mammalian histone deacetylase. *J. Biol. Chem.* 1993, 268, 22429-22435.

[132] Furumai R, Komatsu Y, Nishino N, Khochbin S, Yoshida M, Horinouchi S. Potent histone deacetylase inhibitors built from trichostatin A and cyclic tetrapeptide antibiotics including trapoxin. *Proc. Natl. Acad. Sci. USA* 2001, 98, 87-92.

[133] Jóna A, Khaskhely N, Buglio D, Shafer JA, Derenzini E, Bollard CM, Medeiros LJ, Illés A, Ji Y, Younes A. The histone deacetylase inhibitor entinostat (SNDX-275) induces apoptosis in Hodgkin lymphoma cells and synergizes with Bcl-2 family inhibitors. *Exp. Hematol.* 2011, 39, 1007-1017.

[134] Shen L, Ciesielski M, Ramakrishnan S, Miles KM, Ellis L, Sotomayor P, Shrikant P, Fenstermaker R, Pili R. Class I histone deacetylase inhibitor entinostat suppresses regulatory T cells and enhances immunotherapies in renal and prostate cancer models. *PLOS One* 2012, 7, e30815.

[135] Boumber Y[1], Younes A, Garcia-Manero G. Mocetinostat (MGCD0103): a review of an isotype-specific histone deacetylase inhibitor. *Expert Opin. Investig. Drugs* 2011, 20, 823-829.

[136] Younes A, Oki Y, Bociek RG, Kuruvilla J, Fanale M, Neelapu S, Copeland A, Buglio D, Galal A, Besterman J, Li Z, Drouin M, Patterson T, Ward MR, Paulus JK, Ji Y, Medeiros LJ, Martell RE. Mocetinostat for relapsed classical Hodgkin's lymphoma: an open-label, single-arm, phase 2 trial. *Lancet Oncol.* 2011, 12, 1222-1228.

[137] Santo L, Hideshima T, Kung AL, Tseng JC, Tamang D, Yang M, Jarpe M, van Duzer JH, Mazitschek R, Ogier WC, Cirstea D, Rodig S, Eda H, Scullen T, Canavese M, Bradner J, Anderson KC, Jones SS, Raje N. Preclinical activity, pharmacodynamic, and pharmacokinetic properties

of a selective HDAC6 inhibitor, ACY-1215, in combination with bortezomib in multiple myeloma. *Blood* 2012, 119, 2579-2589.

[138] Gradilone SA, Habringer S, Masyuk TV, Howard BN, Masyuk AI, Larusso NF. HDAC6 is overexpressed in cystic cholangiocytes and its inhibition reduces cystogenesis. *Am. J. Pathol.* 2014, 184, 600-608.

[139] Zhang L, Liu C, Wu J, Tao JJ, Sui XL, Yao ZG, Xu YF, Huang L, Zhu H, Sheng SL, Qin C. Tubastatin A/ACY-1215 improves cognition in Alzheimer's disease transgenic mice. *J. Alzheimers Dis.* 2014, 41, 1193-1205.

[140] el-Beltagi HM, Martens AC, Lelieveld P, Haroun EA, Hagenbeek A. Acetyldinaline: a new oral cytostatic drug with impressive differential activity against leukemic cells and normal stem cells-preclinical studies in a relevant rat model for human acute myelocytic leukemia. *Cancer Res.* 1993, 53, 3008-3014.

[141] Loprevite M, Tiseo M, Grossi F, Scolaro T, Semino C, Pandolfi A, Favoni R, Ardizzoni A. In vitro study of CI-994, a histone deacetylase inhibitor, in non-small cell lung cancer cell lines. *Oncol. Res.* 2005, 15, 39-48.

[142] Hubeek I, Comijn EM, Van der Wilt CL, Merriman RL, Padron JM, Kaspers GJ, Peters GJ. CI-994 (N-acetyl-dinaline) in combination with conventional anti-cancer agents is effective against acute myeloid leukemia in vitro and in vivo. *Oncol. Rep.* 2008, 19, 1517-1523.

[143] Ning ZQ, Li ZB, Newman MJ, Shan S, Wang XH, Pan DS, Zhang J, Dong M, Du X, Lu XP. Chidamide (CS055/HBI-8000): a new histone deacetylase inhibitor of the benzamide class with antitumor activity and the ability to enhance immune cell-mediated tumor cell cytotoxicity. *Cancer Chemother. Pharmacol.* 2012, 69, 901-909.

[144] Davie JR. Inhibition of histone deacetylase activity by butyrate. *J. Nutr.* 2003, 133 (7 Suppl.), 2485S-2493S.

[145] Steliou K, Boosalis MS, Perrine SP, Sangerman J, Faller DV. Butyrate histone deacetylase inhibitors. *Biores. Open Axess* 2012, 1, 192-198.

[146] Bultman SJ. Molecular pathways: gene-environment interactions regulating dietary fiber induction of proliferation and apoptosis via butyrate for cancer prevention. *Clin. Cancer Res.* 2014, 20, 799-803.

[147] Gore SD, Carducci MA. Modifying histones to tame cancer: clinical development of sodium phenylbutyrate and other histone deacetylase inhibitors. *Expert Opin. Investig. Drugs* 2000, 9, 2923-2934.

[148] Kulp SK, Chen CS, Wang DS, Chen CY, Chen CS. Antitumor effects of a novel phenylbutyrate-based histone deacetylase inhibitor, (S)-HDAC-42, in prostate cancer. *Clin. Cancer Res.* 2006, 12, 5199-5206.

[149] Iannitti T, Palmieri B. Clinical and experimental applications of sodium phenylbutyrate. *Drugs R D.* 2011, 11, 227-249.

[150] Phiel CJ, Zhang F, Huang EY, Guenther MG, Lazar MA, Klein PS. Histone deacetylase is a direct target of valproic acid, a potent anticonvulsant, mood stabilizer, and teratogen. *J. Biol. Chem.* 2001, 276, 36734-36741.

[151] Göttlicher M, Minucci S, Zhu P, Krämer OH, Schimpf A, Giavara S, Sleeman JP, Lo Coco F, Nervi C, Pelicci PG, Heinzel T. Valproic acid defines a novel class of HDAC inhibitors inducing differentiation of transformed cells. *EMBO J.* 2001, 20, 6969-6978.

[152] Gurvich N, Tsygankova OM, Meinkoth JL, Klein PS. Histone deacetylase is a target of valproic acid-mediated cellular differentiation. *Cancer Res.* 2004, 64, 1079-1086.

[153] Cipro Š, Hřebačková J, Hraběta J, POljaková J, EcksChlager T. Valproic acid overcomes hypoxia-induced resistance to apoptosis. *Oncol. Rep.* 2012, 27. 1219-1226.

[154] Činčárová L, Zdráhal Z, Fajkus L. New perspectives of valproic acid in clinical practice. *Expert Opin. Investig. Drugs* 2013, 22, 1535-1547.

[155] Hassig CA, Symons KT, Guo X, Nguyen PM, Annable T, Wash PL, Payne JE, Jenkins DA, Bonnefous C, Trotter C, Wang Y, Anzola JV, Milkova EL, Hoffman TZ, Dozier SJ, Wiley BM, Saven A, Malecha JW, Davis RL, Muhammad J, Shiau AK, Noble SA, Rao TS, Smith ND, Hager JH. KD5170, a novel mercaptoketone-based histone deacetylase inhibitor that exhibits broad spectrum antitumor activity in vitro and in vivo. *Mol. Cancer Ther.* 2008, 7, 1054-1065.

[156] Feng R, Ma H, Hassig CA, Payne JE, Smith ND, Mapara MY, Hager JH, Lentzsch S. KD5170, a novel mercaptoketone-based histone deacetylase inhibitor, exerts antimyeloma effects by DNA damage and mitochondrial signaling. *Mol. Cancer Ther.* 2008, 7, 1494-1055.

[157] Payne JE, Bonnefous C, Hassig CA, Symons KT, Guo X, Nguyen PM, Annable T, Wash PL, Hoffman TZ, Rao TS, Shiau AK, Malecha JW, Noble SA, Hager JH, Smith ND. Identification of KD5170: a novel mercaptoketone-based histone deacetylase inhibitor. *Bioorg. Med. Chem. Lett.* 2008, 18, 6093-6096.

[158] Haggarty SJ, Koeller KM, Wong JC, Grozinger CM, Schreiber SL. Domain-selective small-molecule inhibitor of histone deacetylase 6

(HDAC6)-mediated tubulin deacetylation. *Proc. Natl. Acad. Sci. USA* 2003, 100, 4389-4394.

[159] Namdar M, Perez G, Ngo L, Marks PA. Selective inhibition of histone deacetylase 6 (HDAC6) induces DNA damage and sensitizes transformed cells to anticancer agents. *Proc. Natl. Acad. Sci. USA* 2010, 107, 20003-20008.

[160] Aldana-Masangkay GI, Rodriguez-Gonzalez A, Lin T, Ikeda AK, Hsieh YT, Kim YM, Lomenick B, Okemoto K, Landaw EM, Wang D, Mazitschek R, Bradner JE, Sakamoto KM. Tubacin suppresses proliferation and induces apoptosis of acute lymphoblastic leukemia cells. *Leuk. Lymphoma* 2011, 52, 1544-1555.

[161] Souto JA, Vaz E, Lepore I, Pöppler AC, Franci G, Alvarez R, Altucci L, de Lera AR. Synthesis and biological characterization of the histone deacetylase inhibitor largazole and C7- modified analogues. *J. Med. Chem.* 2010, 53, 4654-4667.

[162] Benelkebir H, Marie S, Hayden AL, Lyle J, Loadman PM, Crabb SJ, Packham G, Ganesan A. Total synthesis of largazole and analogues: HDAC inhibition, antiproliferative activity and metabolic stability. *Bioorg. Med. Chem.* 2011, 19, 3650-3658.

[163] Guerra-Bubb JM, Bowers AA, Smith WB, Paranal R, Estiu G, Wiest O, Bradner JE, Williams RM. Synthesis and HDAC inhibitory activity of isosteric thiazoline-oxazole largazole analogs. *Bioorg. Med. Chem. Lett.* 2013, 23, 6025-6028.

[164] Yoshida M, Kijima M, Akita M, Beppu T. Potent and specific inhibition of mammalian histone deacetylase both in vivo and in vitro by trichostatin A. *J. Biol. Chem.* 1990, 265, 17174-17179.

[165] Mann BS, Johnson JR, Cohen MH, Justice R, Pazdur R. FDA approval summary: vorinostat for treatment of advanced primary cutaneous T-cell lymphoma. *Oncologist* 2007, 12, 1247-1252.

[166] Shi B, Xu W. The development and potential clinical utility of biomarkers for HDAC inhibitors. *Drug Disc. Ther.* 2013, 7, 129/136.

[167] Prince HM, Dickinson M, Khot A. Romidepsin for cutaneous T-cell lymphoma. *Future Oncol.* 2013, 9, 1819-1827.

[168] Choudhary C, Kumar C, Gnad F, Nielsen ML, Rehman M, Walther TC, Olsen JV, Mann M. Lysine acetylation targets protein complexes and co-regulates major cellular functions. *Science* 2009, 325, 834-840.

[169] Robert T, Vanoli F, Chiolo I, Shubassi G, Bernstein KA, Rothstein R, Botrugno OA, Parazzoli D, Oldani A, Minucci S, Foiani M. HDACs link

the DNA damage response, processing of double-strand breaks and autophagy. *Nature* 2011, 471, 74-79.

[170] Robert C, Rassool FV. HDAC inhibitors: roles of DNA damage and repair. *Adv. Cancer Res.* 2012, 116, 87-129.

[171] Cornago M, Garcia-Alberich C, Blasco-Angulo N, Vall-Llaura N, Nager M, Herreros J, Comella JX, Sanchis D, Llovera M. Histone deacetylase inhibitors promote glioma cell death by G2 checkpoint abrogation leading to mitotic catastrophe. *Cell Death Dis.* 2014, 5, e1435.

[172] Kaufman JL, Fabre C, Lonial S, Richardson PG. Histone deacetylase inhibitors in multiple myeloma: rationale and evidence for their use in combination therapy. *Clin. Lymphoma Myeloma Leuk.* 2013, 13, 370-376.

[173] Li Z, Zhu WG. Targeting histone deacetylases for cancer therapy: from molecular mechanisms to clinical implications. *Int. J. Biol. Sci.* 2014, 10, 757-770.

[174] Frew AJ, Johnstone RW, Bolden JE. Enhancing the apoptotic and therapeutic effects of HDAC inhibitors. *Cancer Lett.* 2009, 280, 125-133.

[175] Chen S, Dai Y, Pei XY, Grant S. Bim upregulation by histone deacetylase inhibitors mediates interactions with the Bcl-2 antagonist ABT-737: Evidence for distinct roles for Bcl-2, Bcl-xL, and Mcl-1. *Mol. Cell. Biol.* 2009, 29, 6149-6169.

[176] Dong LH, Cheng S, Zheng Z, Wang L, Shen Y, Shen ZX, Chen SJ, Zhao WL. Histone deacetylase inhibitor potentiated the ability of mTOR inhibitor to induce autophagic cell death in Burkitt leukemia/lymphoma. *J. Hematol. Oncol.* 2013, 6, 53

[177] Zhang J, Zhong Q. Histone deacetylase inhibitors and cell death. *Cell. Mol Life Sci.* 2014, 71, 3885-3901.

[178] Oehme I, Linke JP, Böck BC, Milde T, Lodrini M, Hartenstein B, Wiegand I, Eckert C, Roth W, Kool M, Kaden S, Gröne HJ, Schulte JH, Lindner S, Hamacher-Brady A, Brady NR, Deubzer HE, Witt O. Histone deacetylase 10 promotes autophagy-mediated cell survival. *Proc. Natl. Acad. Sci. USA* 2013, 110, E2592-E2601.

[179] Chen S, Sang N. Histone deacetylase inhibitors: the epigenetic therapeutics that repress hypoxia-inducible factors. *J. Biomed. Biotechnol.* 2011, 2011, 197946.

[180] Kang FW, Que L, Wu M, Wang ZL, Sun J. Effects of trichostatin A on HIF-1α and VEGF expression in human tongue squamous cell carcinoma cells in vitro. *Oncol. Rep.* 2012, 28, 193-199.

[181] Brodská B, Holoubek A. Generation of reactive oxygen species during apoptosis induced by DNA-damaging agents and/or histone deacetylase inhibitors. *Oxid. Med. Cell Longev.* 2011, 2011, 253529.

[182] You BR, Park WH. Trichostatin A induces apoptotic cell death of HeLa cells in a Bcl-2 and oxidative stress-dependent manner. *Int. J. Oncol.* 2013, 42, 359-366.

[183] Bali P, Pranpat M, Bradner J, Balasis M, Fiskus W, Guo F, Rocha K, Kumaraswamy S, Boyapalle S, Atadja P, Seto E, Bhalla K. Inhibition of histone deacetylase 6 acetylates and disrupts the chaperone function of heat shock protein 90: a novel basis for antileukemia activity of histone deacetylase inhibitors. *J. Biol. Chem.* 2005, 280, 26729-26734.

[184] Newbold A, Matthews GM, Bots M, Cluse LA, Clarke CJ, Banks KM, Cullinane C, Bolden JE, Christiansen AJ, Dickins RA, Miccolo C, Chiocca S, Kral AM, Ozerova ND, Miller TA, Methot JL, Richon VM, Secrist JP, Minucci S, Johnstone RW. Molecular and biologic analysis of histone deacetylase inhibitors with diverse specificities. *Mol. Cancer Ther.* 2013, 12, 2709-2721.

[185] Park S, Park JA, Kim YE, Song S, Kwon HJ, Lee Y. Suberoylanilide hydroxamic acid induces ROS-mediated cleavage of HSP90 in leukemia cells. *Cell Stress Chaperones* 2014, DOI 10.1007/s12192-014-0533-4.

[186] Rodriguez-Gonzalez A, Lin T, Ikeda AK, Simms-Waldrip T, Fu C, Sakamoto KM. Role of the aggresome pathway in cancer: targeting histone deacetylase 6-dependent protein degradation. *Cancer Res.* 2008, 68, 2557-2560.

[187] Simms-Waldrip T, Rodriguez-Gonzalez A, Lin T, Ikeda AK, Fu C, Sakamoto KM. The aggresome pathway as a target for therapy in hematologic malignancies. *Mol. Genet. Metab.* 2008, 94, 283-286.

[188] Xu WS, Parmigiani RB, Marks PA. Histone deacetylase inhibitors: molecular mechanisms of action. *Oncogene* 2007, 26, 5541-5552.

[189] Tan J, Cang S, Ma Y, Petrillo RL, Liu D. Novel histone deacetylase inhibitors in clinical trials as anti-cancer agents. *J. Hematol. Oncol.* 2010, 3, 5.

[190] Ellis L, Pan Y, Smyth GK, George DJ, McCormack C, Williams-Truax R, Mita M, Beck J, Burris H, Ryan G, Atadja P, Butterfoss D, Dugan M, Culver K, Johnstone RW, Prince HM. Histone deacetylase inhibitor panobinostat induces clinical responses with associated alterations in gene expression profiles in cutaneous T-cell lymphoma. *Clin. Cancer Res.* 2008, 14, 4500-4510.

[191] Momparler RL, Côté S, Momparler LF, Idaghdour Y. Epigenetic therapy of acute myeloid leukemia using 5-aza-2'-deoxycytidine (decitabine) in combination with inhibitors of histone methylation and deacetylation. *Clin. Epigenetics* 2014, 6, 19.

[192] Kirschbaum M, Gojo I, Goldberg SL, Bredeson C, Kujawski LA, Yang A, Marks P, Frankel P, Sun X, Tosolini A, Eid JE, Lubiniecki GM, Issa JP. A phase 1 clinical trial of vorinostat in combination with decitabine in patients with acute myeloid leukaemia or myelodysplastic syndrome. *Brit. J. Haematol.* 2014, 167, 185-193.

[193] Quan P, Moinfar F, Kufferath I, Absenger M, Kueznik T, Denk H, Zatloukal K, Haybaeck J. Effects of targeting endometrial stromal sarcoma cells via histone deacetylase and PI3K/AKT/mTOR signaling. *Anticancer Res.* 2014, 34, 2883-2897.

[194] Abaza MS, Bahman AM, Al-Attiyah RJ. Valproic acid, an anti-epileptic drug and a histone deacetylase inhibitor, in combination with proteasome inhibitors exerts antiproliferative, pro-apoptotic and chemosensitizing effects in human colorectal cancer cells: underlying molecular mechanisms. *Int. J. Mol. Med.* 2014, 34, 513-532.

[195] Burke MJ, Lamba JK, Pounds S, Cao X, Ghodke-Puranik Y, Lindgren BR, Weigel BJ, Verneris MR, Miller JS. A therapeutic trial of decitabine and vorinostat in combination with chemotherapy for relapsed/refractory acute lymphoblastic leukemia. *Am. J. Hematol.* 2014, 89, 889-895.

[196] Berenson JR, Hilger JD, Yellin O, Boccia RV, Matous J, Dressler K, Ghazal HH, Jamshed S, Kingsley EC, Harb WA, Noga SJ, Nassir Y, Swift RA, Vescio R. A phase 1/2 study of oral panobinostat combined with melphalan for patients with relapsed or refractory multiple myeloma. *Ann. Hematol.* 2014, 93, 89-98.

[197] Dimopoulos M, Siegel DS, Lonial S, Qi J, Hajek R, Facon T, Rosinol L, Williams C, Blacklock H, Goldschmidt H, Hungria V, Spencer A, Palumbo A, Graef T, Eid JE, Houp J, Sun L, Vuocolo S, Anderson KC. Vorinostat or placebo in combination with bortezomib in patients with multiple myeloma (VANTAGE 088): a multicentre, randomised, double-blind study. *Lancet Oncol.* 2013, 14, 1129-1140.

[198] Subramanian S, Bates SE, Wright JJ, Espinoza-Delgado I, Piekarz RL. Clinical toxicities of histone deacetylase inhibitors. *Pharmaceuticals* 2010, 3, 2751-2767.

[199] Gaymes TJ, Padus RA, Pla M, Orr S, Omidvar N, Chomienne C, Mufti GJ, Rassool FV. Histone deacetylase inhibitors (HDI) cause DNA damage in leukemia cells: a mechanism for leukemia-specific HDI-dependent apoptosis? *Mol. Cancer Res.* 2006, 4, 563-573.

[200] Grant S. Targeting leukemia stem cells with HDAC inhibitors and modulators of the DNA damage response. *Leukemia Suppl.* 2014, 3, S14-S15.

In: Histone Deacetylase Inhibitors (HDIs)
Editor: Beverly D. Carson
ISBN: 978-1-63463-835-7

Chapter 2

Histone Deacetylase Inhibitors in the Treatment of Lymphoid Malignancies

*Ota Fuchs**
Institute of Hematology and Blood Transfusion
Prague, Czech Republic

Abstract

Histone deacetylase inhibitors (HDACIs) are currently used in the clinic for the treatment of solid and hematological malignancies. In particular, vorinostat (Zolinza) and romidepsin (Istodax) have been approved by the US Food and Drug Administration for the treatment of relapsed and refractory cutaneous T-cell lymphomas (CTCL) patients who have received one or more prior systemic therapy and patients with peripheral T-cell lymphoma (PTCL) who have also received one or more prior therapy. CTCL is the disease with the highest clinical response rates with HDACIs.

Therefore, the studies of the molecular basis of this responsiveness were done in CTCL. At least 35 CpG islands were hypermethylated in tumor stage CTCL samples including that of the putative tumor suppressor gene BCL-7a (B-cell CLL/Lymphoma 7) in 48% of samples. BCL-7, which is located on chromosome 12q 24.31, has been cloned as

* Correspondence: Ota Fuchs, PhD, Tel: 420 221977512; Fax: 420 221977370, E-mail: Ota.Fuchs@uhkt.cz.

part of the chromosomal translocations in Burkitt's lymphoma and is at a site of frequent breakpoints in lymphomas. Further hypermethylated genes can be grouped into cell cycle desregulation (p15, p16 and p73), defective DNA repair gene MGMT (O-6- methylguanine-DNA methyltransferase), apoptosis dysregulation (TMS1 /Target of Methylation- mediated Silencing/ and p73) and chromosomal instability (G2/M checkpoint regulator gene CHFR). p73 is responsible for activation of induced death of T- cells and its silencing leads to accumulation of T cells in tissues, an important step in the pathogenesis of CTCL. Hypermethylation of p73 has also been described in nodal B-cell and NK-cell lymphomas. HDACIs block cell proliferation and cause apoptosis by altering the expression of proteins (cyclins, cyclin dependent kinase inhibitors) involved in growth control.

There is increasing evidence that HDACIs also affect several pathways that are important in cell proliferation and differentiation of lymphoid cells, including the TGF beta pathway, the JAK-STAT pathway, myc and Bcl-6. HDACIs induce death of tumor cells through the induction of both the internal and external pathways of apoptosis, as well as through non-apoptotic mechanisms like autophagy. HDACIs have anti-angiogenic effects.

Presently, there are no HDACIs that are approved for the treatment of B- cell lymphomas. The clinical data of HDACIs in non-Hodgkin lymphomas, mantle cell lymphoma and diffuse large B-cell lymphoma (DLBCL), are promising. High nuclear expression of HDAC2 may play an important role in survival of DLBCL patients. Several HDAC molecules are overexpressed in T-cell and B-cell lymphoid malignancies. STAT family of transcription factors (particularly STAT3 and STAT6) are activated in Hodgkin lymphoma. STAT regulation involves phosphorylation and lysine acetylation. HDACIs could play an important role also in Hodgkin lymphoma. Combinations of HDACIs with hypomethylating agents can also influence antitumor immune responses in Hodgkin lymphoma. The anticancer effects of HDACIs require the immune system. HDACIs are under intense investigation in multiple myeloma. The pro-apoptotic and cell cycle arresting properties are the best characterized features of HDACIs. Among the pleiotropic effects of HDACIs, the proteasome system is also affected and the decreased activity of the 20S proteasome and downregulation of members of ubiquitination-proteasome pathway in multiple myeloma were shown. HDACIs also affect the bone marrow microenvironment. Combinations of HDACIs and proteasome inhibitors have synergistic anticancer effect in multiple myeloma cells.

Keywords: Acetylation, apoptosis, cell cycle, histone deacetylates, HDAC inhibitors, B-cell lymphoma, T-cell lymphoma, multiple myeloma

INTRODUCTION

Trichostatin A (TSA) was the first natural hydroxamate found as HDACs inhibitor [1]. Vorinostat (suberoylanilide hydroxamic acid, Zolinza), which is structurally similar to TSA, was the first HDACI approved on October 6, 2006 by the United States Food and Drug Administration (FDA) for the treatment of relapsed and refractory cutaneous T-cell lymphoma (CTCL) [2]. Resminostat (RAS2410) was approved by the US FDA on Septeber 6, 2011 for patients with Hodgkin's lymphoma [3]. Romidepsin, structurally unique, potent, bicyclic class selective histone deacetylase inhibitor (HDACI), was approved by the US FDA for patients with cutaneous T-cell lymphoma (CTCL) who had received at least one prior systemic therapy and patients with peripheral T-cell lymphoma (PTCL) who had received at least one prior therapy [4]. HDACI romidepsin has demonstrated durable clinical responses and tolerability in patients with relapsed/refractory PTCL and CTCL [5-7]. US FDA approved Beleodaq (belinostat) for patients with relapsed/refractory PTCL on July 3, 2014 [8].

Selection of novel drug therapies for patients with relapsed/refractory aggressive lymphoma requires not only considerations regarding efficacy but also careful evaluation of toxicities as well as overall clinical benefit [9]. Initially HDACIs were developed with the idea that they affected transcriptional activation by modulating chromatin condensation and decondensation. It is now clear that their effects go beyond chromatin and they modify gene expression and cellular function via multiple pathways [10, 11].

Lymphoma is the most common blood cancer. The two main forms of lymphoma are Hodgkin's lymphoma (HL) and non-Hodgkin's lymphoma (NHL). Lymphoma occurs when cells of the immune system called lymphocytes, a type of white blood cell, grow and multiply uncontrollably. Cancerous lymphocytes can travel to many parts of the body, including the lymph nodes, spleen, bone marrow, blood, or other organs, and form a mass called a tumor. The body has two main types of lymphocytes that can develop into lymphomas: B-lymphocytes (B-cells) and T-lymphocytes (T-cells). NHLs comprise a large heterogenous group of lymphoid neoplasms that originate from either mature or immature B-cells, T-cells or natural killer cells [12].

The World Health Organization (WHO) 2008 classification of hematological malignancies defines PTCLs as lymphoid neoplasms originating from mature post-thymic T-cells. PTCLs are diverse with distinct biological subtypes and variable clinical behavior.

CTCL is an epidermotropic form of NHLs caused by mutation of T-cells. The most common forms are Mycosis Fungoides and Sezary Syndrome. The incidence of CTCL in United States increased from 2.8 per million in 1973-1977 to 9.6 per million in 1998-2002; the incidence has since remained steady [13, 14]. As the etiology of CTCL is unknown, the reasons behind this dramatic rise are unknown, but may include improved detection or an increase in exposure to underlying etiologic agents. A new CTCL classification scheme was introduced in 2005, though this should not have affected overall CTCL incidence [15]. Instead, the recent leveling off in incidence may relate to a plateauing of former improvements in physician detection or a stabilization of exposure to etiologic agents. Several European studies have identified associations between CTCL incidence and environmental exposures [16, 17]. US-based studies have reported conflicting results regarding the association between CTCL incidence and both environmental exposures [18-20] and geographic residence [13, 21]. Discrepancies may be attributable to occupational mobility and geographic migration, complicating history of lifetime exposures.

Diffuse large B-cell lymphoma (DLBCL) is the most common type of B-cell lymphoma, accounting for 30-40% of newly diagnosed NHLs [22]. DLBCL involves recurrent translocations of the IGH gene and the deregulation of rearranged oncogenes.

Hodgkin's lymphoma (HL) is divided into two major types, as well as subtypes, according to how the lymph cells look under a microscope and how many Reed-Sternberg cells are present. The epidemiology of HL has heterogeneous characteristics of presentation. HL is an uncommon neoplasm of B-cell origin with an incidence that varies significantly by age, sex, ethnicity, geographic location and socioeconomic status.

In T-cell lymphoma, and Hodgkin lymphoma, increased expression of HDACs in comparison with normal tissues has been observed. This increased HDAC expression correlated with a more aggressive disease course and poorer treatment outcomes [23-25]. Other epigenetic markers were also deregulated in CTCL. Van Doorn and colleagues compared genome wide DNA methylation screening in samples of CTCL with benign skin disorders [26, 27]. They showed widespread promoter hypermethylation in malignant T cells in CTCL, suggesting epigenetic instability. There were hypermethylated promoters of genes involved in cell cycle regulation (*p15, p16, p73*), defective DNA repair genes (O-6-methylguanine-DNA methyltransferase gene, *MGMT*), apoptosis deregulation (tumor suppressor gene, *TMS1*), and chromosomal instability (E3 ubiquitin-protein ligase CHFR / checkpoint with forkhead and ring finger domains/ gene, *CHFR*). This gene (*CHFR*) encodes an E3 ubiquitin-protein ligase required for the maintenance of the antephase checkpoint that regulates cell cycle entry into mitosis and, therefore, may play a key role in cell cycle progression and tumorigenesis. The encoded protein has an N-terminal forkhead-associated domain, a central RING-finger domain, and a cysteine-rich C terminal region.

In contrast with lymphomas, there are no studies showing abnormal expression of HDACs in plasma cell malignancies like myeloma, an mostly incurable B-cell neoplasm. In spite of this, several HDACIs have shown antimyeloma activity [28-34]. The mechanism of this activity remains unclear but may be related to the general effects of HDACIs on cell biology, like upregulation of $p21^{CIP1/WAF1}$, cell cycle arrest, or apoptosis [35-37].

HDACIs in B Cell Lymphoma

Although there is a strong rationale for the use of HDACI in B-cell malignancies, no HDACIs were approved specifically for the treatment of B-cell lymphomas. High nuclear expression of HDAC2 may play an important role in survival of DLBCL patients, especially in those with nodal lymphoma, which is associated with a shorter survival time [22]. B-cell lymphoma 6 protein (BCL6) is a protein that in humans is encoded by the *BCL6* gene [38]. BCL6 is a zinc finger transcription factor and contains an N-terminal POZ (poxvirus and zinc finger) domain. This protein acts as a sequence-specific repressor of transcription, and has been shown to modulate the transcription of START-dependent IL-4 responses of B cells. *IL-4 starts* these B cells into the cell cycle. BCL6 can interact with a variety of POZ-containing proteins that function as transcription corepressors. *BCL6* is found to be frequently translocated and hypermutated in DLBCL, and may be involved in the pathogenesis of DLBCL. The effects of HDACIs on BCL6 provide a rationale for the use of HDACIs either alone or in combination with other agents in cases of lymphoma in which BCL6 is overexpressed [39].

Hypoxia inducible factor (HIF) is important in cancer, as it regulates various oncogenic genes as well as genes involved in cell survival, proliferation, and migration. Elevated HIF-1 protein promotes a more aggressive tumor phenotype, and greater HIF-1 expression has been demonstrated to correlate with poorer prognosis, increased risk of metastasis and increased mortality. Recent reports suggest that HIF-1 activates autophagy, a lysosomal degradation pathway which may promote tumor cell survival. HIF-1α expression is constitutively active in multiple DLBCL cell lines under normoxia and it is regulated by the PI3K/AKT pathway [40]. Abexinostat (PCI-24781), a pan histone HDACI, enhanced accumulation of HIF-1α and induced autophagy initially, while extended incubation with the drug resulted in inhibition of HIF-1α [40]. The hypothesis that PCI-24781-induced autophagy is mediated by HIF-1α and that inhibition of HIF-1α in these cells results in attenuation of autophagy and decreased survival was tested [40]. Evidence that autophagy serves as a survival pathway in DLBCL cells treated with PCI-24781 was provided. This suggests that the use of autophagy inhibitors such as chloroquine or 3-methyl adenine in combination with PCI-24781 may enhance apoptosis in lymphoma cells.

Mantle cell lymphoma (MCL) is a rare, B-cell NHL that most often affects men over the age of 60. The disease may be aggressive (fast growing) but it can also behave in a more indolent (slow growing) fashion in some patients. MCL comprises about five percent of all NHLs. The disease is called “mantle cell lymphoma” because the tumor cells originally come from the “mantle zone” of the lymph node. MCL is usually diagnosed as a late-stage disease that has typically spread to the gastrointestinal tract and bone marrow. Overproduction of a protein cyclin D1, the t(11;14) translocation and loss of the cyclin-dependent kinases inhibitors $p21^{CIP1/WAF1}$, and $p27^{KIP1}$ is found in more than 90 percent of patients with MCL [41-44]. Two of the most prominent effects of HDACI are the downregulation of cyclin D1 and upregulation of both cyclin-dependent kinases inhibitors ($p21^{CIP1/WAF1}$, and $p27^{KIP1}$) [45]. Although initial rituximab-containing chemotherapies achieve high response rates, indolent B-cell non-Hodgkin lymphoma (B-NHL), such as follicular lymphoma (FL), is still incurable. Therefore, new effective agents with novel mechanisms are anticipated. HDACIs are potent epigenetic agents for the treatment of MCL [46].

In the multicentre phase II study [47], patients with relapsed/refractory indolent B-NHL and MCL received vorinostat 200 mg twice daily for 14 consecutive days in a 21-days cycle until disease progression or unacceptable toxicity occurred. The primary endpoint was overall response rate (ORR) in FL patients and safety and tolerability in all patients. Secondary endpoints included progression-free survival (PFS). Fifty-six eligible patients were enrolled; 50 patients (39 with FL, seven with other B-NHL, and four with MCL) were evaluable for ORR, and 40 patients had received rituximab-containing prior chemotherapeutic regimens. For the 39 patients with FL, the ORR was 49% [95% confidence interval (CI): 32.4, 65.2] and the median PFS was 20 months (95% CI: 11.2, 29.7). Major toxicities were manageable grade

3/4 thrombocytopenia (TCP) and neutropenia. Vorinostat offers sustained antitumour activity in patients with relapsed or refractory FL with an acceptable safety profile. Further investigation of vorinostat for clinical efficacy is warranted.

HDACI-induced TCP was not due to myelosuppression or reduced platelet lifespan, but to decreased platelet release from megakaryocytes [48]. Cultured primary murine megakaryocytes showed reductions in proplatelet extensions after HDACI exposure and a dose-dependent increase in the phosphorylation of myosin light chain 2 (MLC2). Phosphorylation of MLC to phospho-MLC (pMLC) and subsequent proplatelet formation in megakaryocytes is regulated by the Rho-GTPase proteins Rac1, CDC42, and RhoA. Primary mouse megakaryocytes and the human megakaryoblastic cell line Meg-01 showed reductions in Rac1, CDC42, and RhoA protein levels after treatment with HDACIs [48]. It possible to overcome HDACI-induced TCP by administering the mouse-specific thrombopoietin (TPO) mimetic AMP-4, which improved platelet numbers to levels similar to untreated controls. This report [46] provides the first detailed account of the molecular and biologic processes involved in HDACI-mediated TCP. Moreover, preclinical studies provide evidence that dose-limiting TCP induced by HDACIs may be circumvented using a TPO mimetic [48].

HDACIs in T Cell Lymphoma

The peripheral T-cell lymphomas (PTCL) are a rare and heterogeneous group of mature T-cell lymphomas with limited available therapies. The outcome of frontline chemotherapy regimens has been disappointing, with a long-term survival of only 20%-30%. There is an urgent need to optimize induction therapy by incorporating novel agents that target the dysregulated pathways. HDACIs that induce acetylation of histones and enhance apoptosis have shown promising activity.

Romidepsin (FK228; previously depsipeptide), an HDACI isolated from *Chromobacterium violaceum* [49, 50], was approved by the US FDA for the treatment of PTCL in patients who have received at least one prior therapy. In a phase II study of romidepsin (14 mg/m^2 administered as a 4- h infusion on days 1, 8 and 15 of a 28-day cycle) in separate cohorts of CTCL and relapsed PTCL patients. The ORR among 45 PTCL patients was 38%, with 18% CR (complete response). Median duration of response was 8.9 months; median duration of CR was 29.7 months. The most common adverse events included nausea, (51%), fatigue (40%), Thrombocytopenia (47%), leukopenia (47%), granulocytopenia (45%), and anemia (40%) [51]. Romidepsin demonstrated clinically meaningful disease control in half of the patients in phase II trial [4-6, 52].

Pharmacokinetics, efficacy, and toxicity of the recently US FDA-approved agent belinostat for its use in patients with relapsed/refractory PTCL was described [8, 53, 54]. Belinostat is a potent hydroxamic acid-derived pan-HDACI [55] that has been evaluated in an phase II studies in patients with relapsed/refractory PTCL. Two phase II studies were completed with belinostat given intravenously in the relapsed/refractory PTCL patients with at least 25% overall response and minimal toxicities [8, 53, 54]. Belinostat demonstrated clinical benefit for patients with refractory or relapsed PTCL in a recent Phase II clinical trial, the BELIEF trial. The evidence available for its use in PTCL is mostly limited to this analysis [8]. This was a single-arm study in which patients with PTCL who had failed at least one prior treatment were eligible for enrollment. The primary study objective was to assess the safety and efficacy of single-agent belinostat in refractory or relapsed PTCL. Inclusion criteria included platelet counts of 50,000/μL or greater, no prior HDACI therapy, and no relapse within 100 days of autologous or allogeneic bone marrow transplant. The primary endpoint was the ORR and secondary endpoints were safety, time to response, progression-free survival, duration of response, and OS. Response by PTCL subtype was also evaluated. Belinostat 1,000 mg/m^2 was administered as a 30-minute intravenous infusion on days 1–5 of a 21-day cycle until disease progression or unacceptable toxicity. There were 129 patients with relapsed or refractory PTCL who received belinostat for a median of two cycles (range 1–33). The population was predominantly male (53%), and the median age was 63 years-old. The majority of patients received CHOP/CHOP-like regimens prior to enrollment (96%), and the median number of systemic therapies was two. A smaller proportion (23%) of patients had previously undergone stem-cell transplantation prior to enrollment. After confirmation of PTCL by central pathology review, there were 120 patients who were eligible for evaluation. Seven patients died prior to first radiologic assessment, ten had clinical progression, five withdrew from the trial, and one was lost to follow up. Twenty-six percent of the remaining patients demonstrated an ORR with 11% having a complete response and 15% a partial response. Stable disease was seen in 15% while 40% had progressive disease. In terms of the three most common subtypes, ORR was seen in 23% of patients with PTCL-NOS (n=77), 46% in AITL (n=22), and 15% in ALCL, ALK-negative (n=13) (0% in ALK-positive [n=2]).

The authors concluded that belinostat can be a novel therapeutic option for patients with low bone marrow reserve and/or thrombocytopenia. Belinostat also demonstrated a possible therapeutic advantage in patients with AITL with a greater ORR and a median progression-free survival of 4.2 months versus 1.6 months seen in all subtypes.

Oral panobinostat, also known as LBH589, is a pan-HDACI belonging to the hydroxamic acid group that has shown remarkable activity in patients with CTCL in a phase I/II trial [9, 56]. Panobinostat was used at a dose of 20 mg a day on a weekly basis.

The activity of romidepsin in CTCL [57] seems to be a class effect, with other HDACI also found to demonstrate activity [58, 59]. Twenty-seven patients were enrolled onto the first cohort, and a total of 71 patients with CTCL are included in this analysis [57]. These patients had undergone a median of four prior treatments, and 62 patients (87%) had advanced-stage disease (stage IIB, n = 15; stage III, n= 6; or stage IV, n = 41). Toxicities included nausea, vomiting, fatigue, and transient thrombocytopenia and granulocytopenia. Pharmacokinetics were evaluated with the first administration of romidepsin. Complete responses were observed in four patients, and partial responses were observed in 20 patients for an overall response rate of 34% (95% CI, 23% to 46%). The median duration of response was 13.7 months. Romidepsin has single-agent clinical activity with significant and durable responses in patients with CTCL. A potent and specific inhibitor of class 1 HDACs, romidepsin has linear pharmacokinetics and is primarily metabolized by cytochrome P-450 isoenzyme 3A4. In two Phase II studies involving patients with relapsed or refractory CTCL, romidepsin therapy produced overall response rates of 34-35% (including patients with advanced and heavily pretreated disease), with a complete response seen in about 6% of patients in both studies; romidepsin responses were seen across all evaluated disease sites (skin, blood, lymph, viscera) [60-63]. Romidepsin had an acceptable tolerability profile, with the most common grade 3 or 4 adverse events considered at least possibly related to romidepsin being hematologic or asthenic in nature.

HDACIs in Hodgkin's Lymphoma

ABVD (doxorubicin, bleomycin, vinblastine, and dacarbazine) regimen has been established as a standard therapy for Hodgkin's lymphoma (HL), and over 70% of patients with HL would be curable. But some refractory diseases still exist. Recent developments of molecular target agents have been expecting to improve the clinical outcomes of HL. Anti CD30 antibody-drug conjugate, brentuximab vedotin, is a promising drug for relapsed and refractory HL, and is also explored to be incorporated into first line therapy. Small molecules such as HDACIs (vorinostat, panobinostat, entinostat, and mocetinostat), PI3-kinase/Akt/mTOR (mammalian target of rapamycin) pathway inhibitors, such as everolimus, as well as lenalidomide and bendamustine, have been proved as active agents for relapsed diseases. Standard care of HL could be changed in next decade by these molecular targeting agents [64].

HDACs alter the transcriptional activities of histones and nonhistone factors, including p53, 17-β-estradiol factor, c-Myc, NF-κB, HIF-1α, heat shock protein 90, TNF-α (tumor necrosis factor α), and TNF receptor apoptosis-inducing ligand. Through these factors, HDACs mediate cell cycle regulation, suppression of apoptosis, modulation of the immune response, suppression of angiogenesis, and regulation of cell motility, proliferation, differentiation, and viability [65, 66]. Many of these pathways are aberrantly expressed in HL [67]; therefore, HDACIs may provide a mechanism to inhibit tumor growth. Additionally, it is known that Hodgkin Reed-Sternberg (HRS) cells, although of B-cell origin, rarely express B-cell antigens. It has been postulated that this phenotypic finding may be epigenetically regulated and therefore potentially reversible [68, 69].

Inhibitors have been synthesized for the zinc-dependent HDAC classes (I, II, and IV), with some agents inhibiting multiple classes and others affecting one individual class or subclass. Over 18 HDACIs are currently in development, with several showing potential activity in HL patients. Both vorinostat and romidepsin are approved for the treatment of cutaneous T-cell lymphomas; however, to date no agent has been approved for the treatment of HL patients [67]. The following HDACIs are currently being tested in heavily pretreated patients with HL.

In vitro studies of the pan-HDACI vorinostat demonstrated apoptosis and evidence of cell cycle arrest in HL cell lines [70]. These findings prompted a phase II trial in 27 heavily pretreated patients. In that study, only one patient had a partial response (PR); however, four others had stable disease (SD) lasting >1 year. Although the ORR was only 4%, treatment was well tolerated and nearly 20% of patients maintained SD or better, leading to additional studies with HDACIs [70].

Panobinostat is an oral pan-HDACI found to be 10 times more potent than vorinostat in cell lines [70, 71]. A phase I/II open-label trial evaluating panobinostat in advanced hematologic malignancies was conducted and antitumor activity was observed in a group of 13 response-evaluable patients with relapsed or refractory HL [70, 71]. Consequently, a phase II study evaluating panobinostat in 129 highly pretreated patients with relapsed HL after autologous stem cell transplant (ASCT) was performed [70]. In total, 41% of patients were refractory to their last therapy and 10% of patients had received an allogeneic SCT. Furthermore, 66% of patients had relapsed within 12 months of their first ASCT. Responses, as measured by computed tomography (CT) or magnetic resonance imaging, were seen in 35 (27%) patients, with five (4%) patients achieving a CR. In addition, 77% of patients had tumor reductions, and the overall duration of response approached 7 months. The median time to response was 7.4 weeks and the median progression-free survival interval was 5.7 months. The estimated 1-year OS rate was 78%, with the median OS time not yet reached. Panobinostat was well tolerated, with grade 3 and 4 toxicities largely confined to cytopenias, which were reversible upon drug interruption or dose reduction [70]. In particular, grade 3 or 4 thrombocytopenia and anemia occurred in 79% and 21% of patients, respectively [70]. Blood counts should initially be evaluated weekly because of the potential for rapid development of cytopenias [70]. The disease control rate of 82% (CR + PR + SD) and the duration of response in a highly treatment refractory population suggest that panobinostat has significant clinical activity in HL treatment. Studies identifying the optimal manner to use panobinostat are under way and include trials investigating the benefit of panobinostat in combination with chemotherapy in the salvage setting [70].

Entinostat is an oral class I isoform-selective HDACI currently being evaluated in an open-label phase II trial in patients with relapsed or refractory HL. Enrollment is ongoing; however, preliminary analysis of 24 patients identified two responding patients (8%). Consistent with findings with other HDACIs, 65% of patients achieved disease control (PR + CR + SD) and toxicities were manageable, with cytopenias predominating [70].

Mocetinostat is a class I and class IV HDACI. Preclinical activity was identified in HL and led to a phase II open-label study in patients with relapsed or refractory disease. In the most recent update, 51 patients were enrolled, with 14 (27%) achieving a PR (n = 12) or CR (n = 2) and one patient achieving durable SD. Grade 3 or higher adverse events (AEs) were notable for cytopenias, abnormal liver function studies, and pericardial effusions [70]. Although mocetinostat showed clinical activity, concerns surrounding the development of nonfatal pericardial effusions have precluded further clinical development in HL patients at this time [72, 73].

Additionally, HDACIs have shown preclinical synergism with a number of other antineoplastic drugs, including hypomethylating agents, conventional chemotherapeutic agents, mTOR inhibitors, and bortezomib, resulting in several ongoing or planned trials aimed to evaluate combinations of HDACIs in an effort to improve these results [64, 74-76].

The HRS cells of classical Hodgkin lymphoma (HL) are surrounded by a number of reactive and inflammatory cells [77]. The ability of HRS cells to evade immune surveillance is linked to a network of cytokines and chemokines that are produced by HRS and the surrounding cells, in addition to the occasional aberrant expression of programmed death ligand-1 (PDL-1) by HRS that inhibits the activation of PD1-expressing T lymphocytes. HDACIs can alter the levels of cytokines and chemokines *in vitro*, favoring a TH1-type immune response [77]. HDACIs also enhance antitumor immunity by HDAC11-mediated upregulation of OX40 (CD134) ligand (OX40L;CD252) [78]. Both, OX40 and OX40L are members of the tumor necrosis factor receptor/tumor necrosis factor superfamily and are expressed on activated CD4(+) and CD8(+) T cells as well as on a number of other lymphoid and non-lymphoid cells.

Panobinostat induces cell death, autophagy and increase the expression of natural killer cell receptors in HL cell lines [70, 71, 79]. It triggers an enhanced lymphocyte-dependent lyses of HL cells, suppresses the IFN-gamma release and increases TNF-alpha secretion [79]. A recent phase II study of panobinostat in 129 patients with relapsed or refractory HL showed overall response rate of 27% including complete response in 4% [80]. Tumor size reduction was observed in 74% of patients, and the median progression-free survival duration was 6.1 months [80].

In a subset of patients in this study, several serum cytokine and chemokine levels were analyzed, and the decrease of early thymus and activation-regulated chemokine (TARC) levels were found associated with clinical responses [81].

The present study shows the *in vivo* effect of the pan-HDAC inhibitor panobinostat on an expanded panel of 52 serum cytokines and chemokines from the phase II study. In addition, a pilot study of peripheral blood lymphocytes for PD1 expression before and after panobinostat treatment was conducted.

HDACIs in Acute Lymphoblastic Leukemia

Although most studies have focused on methylation of histones to assess the importance of epigenetics in acute lymphoblastic leukemia (ALL), new studies point to the importance of acetylation as well. In newly diagnosed ALL patients without poor risk cytogenetics a higher level of histone H4 acetylation was associated with increased rates of complete remission, extended relapse-free survival, and better overall survival [82].

Despite some limitations, current studies clearly show that epigenetic modifications in ALL are prevalent and have important pathogenic, prognostic and therapeutic significance. Certainly, epigenetic alterations can be reversed pharmacologically unlike the genetic alterations that are also prevalent in cancer. This exciting prospect has attracted significant research and investment.

The growth inhibitory and apoptogenic potential of the pan-HDACi SAHA and the sub-class I selective HDACI MS275, as well as valproic acid (VPA) on glucocorticoid sensitive and resistant B (B-ALL) and T (T-ALL) cells and patients blasts was compared [83]. In contrast, to previous results with U937 acute myeloid leukemia (AML) cells which showed a similar activity of MS275 and SAHA in growth inhibition and apoptosis induction, both B and T-ALL cells were much more efficiently killed by SAHA and VPA than by MS275. The same relative potency was observed with some patient ALL blasts treated ex vivo. SAHA displayed similar efficacy on glucocorticoid-sensitive and insensitive ALL cells but did not synergize with dexamethasone. In studying mediators of apoptosis we found that the TRAIL receptor DR5 is constitutively expressed in glucocorticoid-sensitive CEM-C7 cells which are also TRAIL sensitive. In contrast, glucocorticoid-insensitive CEM-C1 cells do not express DR5 and are insensitive to TRAIL. However, SAHA induces, in addition to $p21^{(WAF1/CIP1)}$ also re-expression of DR5. Importantly, SAHA-induced apoptosis of CEM-C7 cells operates through initiator caspase 10, while it induces apoptosis of CEM-C1 cells through the intrinsic, as well as through caspase-independent death pathways. These data suggest that the generation of resistance to glucocorticoids has dramatically altered death signaling in these cells and that SAHA overcomes these restrictions by inducing alternative death pathways [83].

In the pediatric population, B-acute lymphoblastic leukemia (B-ALL) is the most prevalent childhood hematological malignancy, as well as the leading cause of childhood cancer-related mortality [84]. The fusion protein TEL-AML1 in t(12;21)+ ALL recruits co-repressors and histone deacetylases

(HDACs), which transrepress AML1 target genes. Normal bone marrow cells were more resistant to HDACI FK228 induced cell killing than were cells from ALL patients with or without t(12;21) [85]. FK228 induced differentiation in ALL, irrespective of the presence of t(12;21) [85].

Tubacin is the HDAC6-selective inhibitor which inhibits alpha-tubulin deacetylation in mammalian cells [86]. HDAC6, a class II HDAC, has two catalytic domains, a ubiquitin-binding zinc-finger domain, and a dynein-binding domain, and selectively deacetylates nonhistone proteins such as tubulin, HSP90, cortactin, and peroxiredoxins. Only one of the two catalytic domains of HDAC6 possesses tubulin deacetylase activity, and only this domain is bound by tubacin. Selective inhibition of HDAC6 can affect a number of cellular pathways important in tumorigenesis. Hyperacetylation of HSP90 in response to HDAC6 inhibition reduces the chaperone association with its client proteins, resulting in polyubiquitination and proteasomal degradation of a number of HSP90 substrates. HDAC6 inhibition enhances α-tubulin acetylation, which stabilizes microtubules and is often associated with reduced cell movement. Through the ubiquitin-binding domain, HDAC6 has been shown to recruit polyubiquitinated proteins to dynein motors and to transport protein cargo to aggresomes. HDAC6 inhibition can abrogate HSP90 chaperone function when combined with the HSP90 inhibitor 17-AAG in human leukemia cells, augment the cytotoxic effects of paclitaxel), and enhance thc cytotoxicity of the proteasome inhibitor bortezomib. Aldana-Masangkay et al. [87] provided important new information regarding the therapeutic potential of HDAC6-inhibition in B- and T-ALL cells in comparison to normal jymphocytes. Apoptosis of ALL cells was associated with rapid acetylation of α-tubulin and accumulation of ubiquitinated proteins. ALL cells treated with tubacin undergo apoptosis through caspase activation but through an SAPK/JNK-signaling pathway and Hsp90-independent pathway. This mechanism is different from inhibition of HDAC6 in muliple myeloma and AML cells by tubacin [87, 88].

HDACIs in Chronic Lymphocytic Leukemia

HDAC isoenzyme levels in chronic lymphocytic leukemia (CLL) were significantly increased in class I including HDAC1 and HDAC3, in class II including HADC6, HDAC7, HDAC9 and HDAC10, and in class III including SIRT1 and SIRT6 [89]. Higher HDAC expression activity may indicate a poor prognosis and more advanced disease stage (through indirect evidence), since higher values were found in patients with ZAP-70 (70-kDa zeta-associated protein, a transducing signaling kinase downstream of the T-cell receptor) + and higher CD44, a cell-surface glycoprotein involved in cell–cell interactions, cell adhesion and migration, expression levels [90, 91]. ZAP-70 expression is associated with increased B-cell receptor (BCR) signaling in CLL cells. ZAP70 is a recognized adverse prognostic marker in CLL, associated with enhanced B-cell receptor signaling, significantly more aggressive disease course and poor overall survival. ZAP70 is ordinarily expressed in T cells where it has a crucial role in T-cell receptor signaling, whereas its aberrant expression in CLL leads to enhanced B-cell receptor signaling and significantly more aggressive disease course.

HDACs play a key role in the regulation of acetylation status not only of histones but also of many other non-histone proteins involved in cell cycle regulation, differentiation or apoptosis. Therefore, HDACI have emerged as promising anticancer agents. The characterization of apoptosis in B-cell CLL induced by two HDACI, Kendine 92 and SAHA was described [92]. Both inhibitors induced dose-, time- and caspase-dependent apoptosis through the mitochondrial pathway. Interestingly, Kendine 92 and SAHA showed a selective cytotoxicity for B lymphocytes and induced apoptosis in CLL cells with mutated or deleted TP53 as effectively as in tumor cells harboring wild-type TP53. The pattern of apoptosis-related gene and protein expression profile has been characterized. It has shown to be irrespective of TP53 status and highly similar between SAHA and Kendine 92 exposure. The balance between the increased pro-apoptotic BAD, BNIP3L, BNIP3, BIM, PUMA and AIF mRNA expression levels, and decreased expression of anti-apoptotic BCL-W, BCL-2, BFL-1, XIAP and FLIP indicates global changes in the apoptosis mRNA expression profile consistent with the apoptotic outcome. Protein expression analysis shows increased levels of pro-apoptotic NOXA, BIM and PUMA proteins upon Kendine 92 and SAHA treatment. Our results highlight the capability of these molecules to induce apoptosis not only in a selective manner but also in those cells frequently resistant to standard treatments. Thus, Kendine 92 is a novel HDACI with anticancer efficacy for non-proliferating CLL cells [92].

The isotype-selective HDACI MGCD0103 treatment in CLL resulted in the activation of a caspase cascade downstream of caspase-9, caspase-dependent amplification of mitochondrial depolarization, activation of calpain, and Bax cleavage [93]. A model whereby the intrinsic pathway of apoptosis triggered by MGCD0103 in CLL is associated with a mitochondrial death amplification loop was proposed [93]. MGCD0103 decreases the autophagic flux in primary CLL cells [94]. Activation of the PI3K/AKT/mTOR pathway, together with the activation of caspases, and to a minor extent CAPN1 (calpain-1 catalytic subunit), resulting in cleavage of autophagy components, were involved in MGCD0103-mediated inhibition of autophagy. In addition, MGCD0103 directly modulated the expression of critical autophagy genes at the transcriptional level that may contribute to autophagy impairment. Besides, it was shown that autophagy is a pro-survival mechanism in CLL. Autophagy disruption potentiates cell death induced by anticancer molecules including HDAC and cyclin-dependent kinase inhibitors. In particular, the data highlight the therapeutic potential of MGCD0103 as not only an inducer of apoptosis but also an autophagy suppressor in both combination regimens with molecules like flavopiridol, known to induce protective autophagy in CLL cells, or as an alternative to circumvent undesired immunomodulatory effects seen in the clinic with conventional autophagy inhibitors [94].

HDACIs in Multiple Myeloma

HDACI have already been evaluated in multiple myeloma (MM) including TSA [95], vorinostat [29, 96], depsipeptide [97], KD5170 [98], NVP-LAQ824 [28], VPA [30, 99], and panobinostat [100]. Histone deacetylase inhibitors induce G1 cell cycle arrest in MMCs through dephosphorylation of retinoblastoma protein and increase expression of p53 and p21 [95, 96, 99]. Histone deacetylase inhibitors induce apoptosis by dowregulation of Bcl-2 family members [96, 97] and overcome drug resistance mediated by the BM environment [96]. Furthermore, glucose-regulated protein 78 (GRP78) was recently identified as a novel non-histone target of HDACIs [101, 102]. Glucose-regulated protein 78 has a central role in the unfolded protein response (UPR). Glucose-regulated protein 78 acetylation following HDACI treatment was described to activate UPR and contributes to the antitumour activity of HDACIs. Class 1 HDACs binding to GRP78, within the endoplasmic reticulum (ER), represent a novel mode of UPR regulation and an interesting mechanism of HDACIs action [103]. The ER of normal PCs and MMCs is well developed to accommodate the production and secretion of large amounts of immunoglobulins. That is why association of HDACIs with proteasome inhibitors could be promising in MM treatment [104]. When used as a single agent in patients with relapsing/refractory MM, HDACIs have shown modest antitumour activity

[105, 106]. In combination with other anti-MM treatments, HDACIs can induce durable antitumour responses [107, 108].

To improve the clinical testing of the efficacy of novel agents, a major stake is identify patients who could benefit from treatment by finding biomarkers predictive for sensitivity of MMCs to HDACIs. We recently reported the development of a gene expression-based risk score predicting the sensitivity of MMCs to DNA methylation inhibitors [109]. In this study, we used the same strategy to build a histone acetylation (HA) score, based on genes whose expression is deregulated by HDACIs in MMCs. Histone acetylation score score makes it possible to identify a subgroup of 42% of patients with short overall survival (OS), whose MMCs are highly sensitive to HDAC inhibition.

Despite the promising preclinical activity of HDACIs in MM cells, their clinical efficacy in monotherapy in relapsed/refractory MM patients was very modest [110]. This promted the development of several combinations among which the one with the strongest scientific rationale is probably that of HDACIs and proteasome inhibitors [107, 108, 111, 112]. The basis is the simultaneous targeting of several mechanisms involved in the UPR. The inhibition of the proteasome blocks the degradation of the ubiquitinated misfolded proteins and the use of HDACIs interferes with the activity of heat-shock proteins, which are necessary for the correct folding of proteins. Inhibition of HDAC6 interferes with aggresome formation and autophagy and is also important for the elimination of toxic misfolded proteins. These events induce the accumulation of toxic misfolded proteins in the MM cells with ineffective UPR, leading to apoptosis [110]. These findings present HDAC6 as an interesting novel target. ACY-1215, a novel, selective, orally bioavailable HDAC6 inhibitor, alone and in combination with bortezomib was tested in MM in preclinical studies [113]. The results of *in vitro* and *in vivo* studiesshow significant and synergistic anti MM activity of ACY-1215 in combination with bortezomib and provide the rationale for advancement of this combination into clinical development.

HDACIs in Waldenström Macroglobulinemia

Waldenström macroglobulinemia (WM) is a low-grade lymphoproliferative disorder characterized by bone marrow infiltration of lymphoplasmacytic cells and the production of monoclonal immunoglobulin (IgM) protein. The safety and activity of the HDACI panobinostat in patients with relapsed/refractory WM was studied [114]. Eligibility criteria included patients with relapsed/refractory WM with any number of prior therapies. Patients received panobinostat at 30 mg 3 times a week; 12 of 36 (33%) patients were enrolled at 25 mg dose. A total of 36 patients received therapy. The median age was 62 years (range, 47-80) and the median number of prior therapies was 3 (range, 1-8). All of the patients had received prior rituximab. Minimal response (MR) or better was achieved in 47% of patients (90% confidence interval [CI], 33-62), with 22% partial remissions and 25% MR. In addition, 18 (50%) patients achieved stable disease and none showed progression while on therapy. The median time to first response was 1.8 months (range, 1.7-3.2). The median progression-free survival was 6.6 months (90% CI, 5.5-14.8). Grade 3 and 4 toxicities included thrombocytopenia (67%), neutropenia (36%), anemia (28%), leukopenia (22%), and fatigue (11%). Therefore, panobinostat is an active therapeutic agent in patients with relapsed/ refractory WM [114].

The mitogen-activated protein kinase (MAPK) pathways consist of a group of evolutionarily conserved signaling cascades that regulate cellular response to a variety of stimuli, including cytokines and environmental stresses. These signaling cascades control diverse cellular processes, including cell survival, proliferation, differentiation, apoptosis, motility, and metabolism. In general, the Ras/Raf/MEK1/2/ERK1/2 cascade promotes cell survival, whereas the stress-related p38 and JNK (c-Jun N-terminal kinase) cascades promote apoptosis. In fact, the relative balance between these pro- and anti-apoptotic signaling pathways is believed to represent a critical determinant of cell survival. To date, relatively little attention has been paid to the impact of HDACIs on stress-related MAPK pathways, although an association between HDACIs-mediated JNK activation and cell death has been described [115]. Another HDACI vorinostat induces a stress response in WM cells which leads to activation of stresss-related members of the MAPK family, while simultaneously disabling the cytoprotective MEK1/2/ERK1/2 pathway, leading to a shift in the net balance away from survival and towards death signaling [116, 117].

Conclusion and Perspectives

HDACIs are a relative new class of anti-cancer agents that play important roles in epigenetic or non-epigenetic regulation. HDACIs induce death, apoptosis, and cell cycle arrest in cancer cells. Current relapsed or refractory patients with hematologic lymphoid malignancies outcomes suggest the need for novel regimens and alternative strategies to improve disease management and extend the duration of response. HDACIs may help to improve patient outcomes. Development of novel therapies is connected with the development of new combinations of these agents with other anti-cancer therapeutics, to improve response rates and durability of responses. For example, the ontogenetic Wnt pathway shows almost no activity in adult tissues. In contrast, CLL cells show constitutionally active Wnt signaling. This results in increased resistance to apoptosis. Trichostatin A effectively induces apoptosis in CLL cells via inhibition of Wnt signaling [118]. Combining Trichostatin A with established CLL drugs fludarabine or bendamustine showed an additive effect *in vitro* [118]. Treatment of CLL cells with HDACI MS-275 activates the transcription from the tumor suppressor gene E-cadherin which is frequently silenced in CLL cells. The re-expressed E-cadherin binds to beta-catenin with inhibition of the active Wnt-beta-catenin pathway in CLL cells [119-121]. Increased mitogenic signaling through activation of the mTOR pathway is a common feature of lymphoid malignancies [122, 123]. Synergy of the mTOR inhibitor sirolimus and the HDACI entinostat was shown in mouse plasmacytoma, human Burkitt's lymphoma and human MM cells [123]. Combination therapies targeting NF-κB signaling pathway, other signaling pathways and using HDACIs in MM have been recently reviewed [124, 125].

ACKNOWLEDGMENTS

This work was supported by research project (Ministry of Health, Czech Republic) for conceptual development of research organization (00023736; Institute of Hematology and Blood Transfusion, Prague).

REFERENCES

[1] Yoshida M, Kijima M, Akita M, Beppu T. Potent and specific inhibition of mammalian histone deacetylase both in vivo and in vitro by trichostatin A. *J. Biol. Chem.* 1990, 265, 17174-17179.

[2] Mann BS, Johnson JR, Cohen MH, Justice R, Pazdur R. FDA approval summary: vorinostat for treatment of advanced primary cutaneous T-cell lymphoma. *Oncologist* 2007, 12, 1247-1252.

[3] Shi B, Xu W. The development and potential clinical utility of biomarkers for HDAC inhibitors. *Drug Disc. Ther.* 2013, 7, 129-136.

[4] Prince HM, Dickinson M, Khot A. Romidepsin for cutaneous T-cell lymphoma. *Future Oncol.* 2013, 9, 1819-1827.

[5] Coiffier B, Pro B, Prince HM, Foss F, Sokol L, Greenwood M, Caballero D, Morschhauser F, Wilhelm M, Pinter-Brown L, Padmanabhan Iyer S, Shustov A, Nielsen T, Nichols J, Wolfson J, Balser B, Horwitz S. Romidepsin for the treatment of relapsed/refractory peripheral T-cell lymphoma: pivotal study update demonstrates durable responses. *J. Hematol. Oncol.* 2014, 7, 11.

[6] Foss F, Coiffier B, Horwitz S, Pro B, Prince HM, Sokol L, Greenwood M, Lerner A, Caballero D, Baran E, Kim E, Nichols J, Balser B, Wolfson J, Whittaker S. Tolerability to romidepsin in patients with relapsed/refractory T-cell lymphoma. *Biomark. Res.* 2014, 2, 16.

[7] Finn N, Larouche JF. Romidepsin used as monotherapy in sequence with allogeneic stem cell transplant in a patient with peripheral T-cell lymphoma. *Case Rep Hematol.* 2014, 2014, 404078.

[8] Bodiford A, Bodqe M, Talbott MS, Reddy NM. Profile of belinostat for the treatment of relapsed or refractory peripheral T-cell lymphoma. *OncoTargets Ther.* 2014, 7, 1971-1977.

[9] Zain J, O'Connor OA. Targeting histone deacetylases in the treatment of B- and T-cell malignancies. *Invest. New Drugs* 2010, 28 (Suppl.1), S58-S78.

[10] Li Z, Zhu WG. Targeting histone deacetylases for cancer therapy: from molecular mechanisms to clinical implications. *Int. J. Biol. Sci.* 2014, 10, 757-770.

[11] Zhang J, Zhong Q. Histone deacetylase inhibitors and cell death. *Cell. Mol. Life Sci.* 2014, 71, 3885-3901.

[12] Hassler MR, Schiefer AI, Egger G. Combating the epigenome: epigenetic drugs against non-Hodgkin's lymphoma. *Epigenomics* 2013, 5, 397-415.

[13] Criscione VD, Weinstock MA. Incidence of cutaneous T-cell lymphoma in the United States, 1973-2002. *Arch. Dermatol.* 2007, 143, 854-859.

[14] Korgavkar K, Xiong M, Weinstock M. Changing incidence trends of cutaneous T-cell lymphoma. *JAMA Dermatol.* 2013, 149, 1295-1299.

[15] Willemze R, Jaffe ES, Burg G, Cerroni L, Berti E, Swerdlow SH, et al. WHO-EORTC classification for cutaneouslymphomas. *Blood* 2005, 105, 768-785.

[16] Morales-Suarez-Varela MM, Olsen J, Johansen P, Kaerlev L, Guenel P, Arveux P, et al. Occupational exposures and mycosis fungoides. A European multicentre case-control study (Europe). *Cancer Causes Control: CCC.* 200, 516, 1253-1259.

[17] Mester B, Nieters A, Deeg E, Elsner G, Becker N, Seidler A. Occupation and malignant lymphoma: a population based case control study in Germany. *Occup. Environm. Med.* 2006, 63, 17-26.

[18] Fischmann AB, Bunn PA, Jr., Guccion JG, Matthews MJ, Minna JD. Exposure to chemicals, physical agents, and biologic agents in mycosis fungoides and the Sezary syndrome. *Cancer Treat. Rep.* 1979, 63, 591-596.

[19] Tuyp E, Burgoyne A, Aitchison T, MacKie R. A case-control study of possible causative factors in mycosis fungoides. *Arch Dermatol.* 1987, 123, 196-200.

[20] Whittemore AS, Holly EA, Lee IM, Abel EA, Adams RM, Nickoloff BJ, et al. Mycosis fungoides in relation to environmental exposures and immune response: a case-control study. *J. Natl. Cancer Inst.* 1989, 81, 1560-1567.

[21] Epstein EH, Jr., Levin DL, Croft JD, Jr., Lutzner MA. Mycosis fungoides. Survival, prognostic features, response to therapy, and autopsy findings. *Medicine (Baltimore).* 1972, 51, 61-72.

[22] Lee SH, Yoo C, Im S, Jung JH, Choi HJ, Yoo J. Expression of histone deacetylases in diffuse large B-cell lymphoma and its clinical significance. *Int. J. Med. Sci.* 2014, 11, 994-1000.

[23] Marquard L, Poulsen CB, Gjerdrum LM, de Nully Brown P, Christensen IJ, Jensen PB, Sehested M, Johansen P, Ralfkiaer E. Histone deacetylase 1, 2, 6 and acetylated histone H4 in B- and T-cell lymphomas. *Histopathology* 2009, 54, 688-698.

[24] Adams H, Fritzsche FR, Dirnhofer S, Kristiansen G, Tzankov A. Class I histone deacetylases 1, 2 and 3 are highly expressed in classical Hodgkin's lymphoma. *Expert. Opin. Ther. Targets* 2010, 14, 577-584.

[25] Zain J. Role of histone deacetylase inhibitors in the treatment of lymphomas and multiple myeloma. *Hematol. Oncol. Clin. N. Am.* 2012, 26, 671-704.

[26] van Doorn R, Gruis NA, Willemze R, van der Velden PA, Tensen CP. Aberrant DNA methylation in cutaneous malignancies. *Semin. Oncol.* 2005, 32, 479-487.

[27] van Doorn R, Zoutman WH, Dijkman R, de Menezes RX, Commandeur S, Mulder AA, van der Velden PA, Vermeer MH, Willemze R, Yan PS,

Huang TH, Tensen CP. Epigenetic profiling of cutaneous T-cell lymphoma: promoter hypermethylation of multiple tumor suppressor genes including BCL7a, PTPRG, and p73. *J. Clin. Oncol.* 2005, 23, 3886-3896.

[28] Catley L, Weisberg E, Tai YT, Atadja P, Remiszewski S, Hideshima T, Mitsiades N, Shringarpure R, LeBlanc R, Chauhan D, Munshi NC, Schlossman R, Richardson P, Griffin J, Anderson KC. NVP-LAQ824 is a potent novel histone deacetylase inhibitor with significant activity against multiple myeloma. *Blood* 2003, 102, 2615-2622.

[29] Mitsiades CS, Mitsiades NS, McMullan CJ, Poulaki V, Shringarpure R, Hideshima T, Akiyama M, Chauhan D, Munshi N, Gu X, Bailey C, Joseph M, Libermann TA, Richon VM, Marks PA, Anderson KC. Transcriptional signature of histone deacetylase inhibition in multiple myeloma: biological and clinical implications. *Proc. Natl. Acad. Sci. U S A* 2004, 101, 540-545.

[30] Kaiser M, Zavrski I, Sterz J, Jakob C, Fleissner C, Kloetzel PM, Sezer O, Heider U. The effects of the histone deacetylase inhibitor valproic acid on cell cycle, growth suppression and apoptosis in multiple myeloma. *Haematologica* 2006, 91, 248-251.

[31] Ocio EM, López-Pérez R, Mateo G, Gutiérrez N, Atadja P, Pandiella A, San Miguel JF. The histone deacetylase inhibitor LBH589 is a potent antimyeloma agent that overcomes drug resistance. *Cancer Res.* 2006, 66, 5781-5789.

[32] Stühmer T, Arts J, Chatterjee M, Borawski J, Wolff A, King P, Einsele H, Leo E, Bargou RC. Preclinical anti-myeloma activity of the novel HDAC-inhibitor JNJ-26481585. *Br. J. Haematol.* 2010, 149, 529-536.

[33] Mandl-Weber S, Meinel FG, Jankowsky R, Oduncu F, Schmidmaier R, Baumann P. The novel inhibitor of histone deacetylase resminostat (RAS2410) inhibits proliferation and induces apoptosis in multiple myeloma (MM) cells. *Br. J. Haematol.* 2010, 149, 518-528.

[34] Baumann P, Junghanns C, Mandl-Weber S, Strobl S, Oduncu F, Schmidmaier R. The pan-histone deacetylase inhibitor CR2408 disrupts cell cycle progression, diminishes proliferation and causes apoptosis in multiple myeloma cells. *Br. J. Haematol.* 2012, 156, 633-642.

[35] Sandor V, Senderowicz A, Mertins S, Sackett D, Sausville E, Blagosklonny MV, Bates SE. P21-dependent g(1)arrest with downregulation of cyclin D1 and upregulation of cyclin E by the histone deacetylase inhibitor FR901228. *Br. J. Cancer* 2000, 83, 817-825.

[36] Marks PA, Richon VM, Rifkind RA. Histone deacetylase inhibitors: inducers of differentiation or apoptosis of transformed cells. *J. Natl. Cancer Inst.* 2000, 92, 1210-1216.

[37] Mita MM, Mita AC, Tolcher AW. Apoptosis: mechanisms and implications for cancer therapeutics. *Targ. Oncol.* 2006, 1, 197-214.

[38] Kawamata N, Miki T, Fukuda T, Hirosawa S, Aoki N. The organization of the BCL6 gene. *Leukemia* 1994, 8, 1327-1330.

[39] Pasqualucci L, Migliazza A, Basso K, Houldsworth J, Chaganti RS, Dalla-Favera R. Mutations of the BCL6 proto-oncogene disrupt its negative autoregulation in diffuse large B-cell lymphoma. *Blood* 2003, 101, 2914-2923.

[40] Bhalla S, Evens AM, Prachand S, Schumacker PT, Gordon LI. Paradoxical regulation of hypoxia inducible factor-1α (HIF-1α) by histone deacetylase inhibitor in diffuse large B-cell lymphoma. *PLoS One* 2013, 8, e81333.

[41] McKay P, Leach M, Jackson R, Cook G, Rule S; British Committee for Standards in Haematology. Guidelines for the investigation and management of mantle cell lymphoma. *Br. J. Haematol.* 2012, 159, 405-426.

[42] Dreyling M, Kluin-Nelemans HC, Beà S, Klapper W, Vogt N, Delfau-Larue MH, Hutter G, Cheah C, Chiappella A, Cortelazzo S, Pott C, Hess G, Visco C, Vitolo U, Klener P, Aurer I, Unterhalt M, Ribrag V, Hoster E, Hermine O; European MCL Network. Update on the molecular pathogenesis and clinical treatment of mantle cell lymphoma: report of the 11th annual conference of the European Mantle Cell Lymphoma Network. *Leuk. Lymphoma* 2013, 54, 699-707.

[43] Zaja F, Federico M, Vitolo U, Zinzani PL. Managenent of relapsed/refractory mantle cell lymphoma: a review of current therapeutic strategies. *Leuk. Lymphoma* 2014, 55, 988-998.

[44] Gordon LI, Bernstein SH, Jares P, Kahl BS, Witzig TE, Dreyling M. Recent advances in mantle cell lymphoma: report of the 2013 mantle cell lymphoma consortium workshop. *Leuk. Lymphoma* 2014, 55, 2262-2270.

[45] Prince HM, Bishton MJ, Harrison SJ. Clinical studies of histone deacetylase inhibitors. *Clin. Cancer Res.* 2009, 15, 3958-3969.

[46] Ghai V, Sharma K, Abbi KK, Shimko S, Epner EM. Current approaches to epigenetic therapy for the treatment of mantle cell lymphoma. *Adv. Exp. Med. Biol.* 2013, 779, 257-266.

[47] Ogura M, Ando K, Suzuki T, Ishizawa K, Oh SY, Itoh K, Yamamoto K, Au WY, Tien HF, Matsuno Y, Terauchi T, Yamamoto K, Mori M, Tanaka Y, Shimamoto T, Tobinai K, Kim WS. A multicentre phase II study of vorinostat in patients with relapsed or refractory indolent B-cell non-Hodgkin lymphoma and mantle cell lymphoma. *Br. J. Haematol.* 2014, 165, 768-776.

[48] Bishton MJ, Harrison SJ, Martin BP, McLaughlin N, James C, Josefsson EC, Henley KJ, Kile BT, Prince HM, Johnstone RW. Deciphering the molecular and biologic processes that mediate histone deacetylase inhibitor-induced thrombocytopenia. *Blood* 2011, 117, 3658-3668.

[49] Ueda H, Nakajima H, Hori Y, Fujita T, Nishimura M, Goto T, Okuhara M. FR901228, a novel antitumor bicyclic depsipeptide produced by Chromobacterium violaceum No. 968. I. Taxonomy, fermentation, isolation, physico-chemical and biological properties, and antitumor activity. *J. Antibiot. (Tokyo)* 1994, 47, 301-310.

[50] Nakajima H, Kim YB, Terano H, Yoshida M, Horinouchi S. FR901228, a potent antitumor antibiotic, is a novel histone deacetylase inhibitor. *Exp. Cell Res.* 1998, 241, 126-133.

[51] Piekarz RL, Frye R, Prince HM, Kirschbaum MH, Zain J, Allen SL, Jaffe ES, Ling A, Turner M, Peer CJ, Figg WD, Steinberg SM, Smith S, Joske D, Lewis I, Hutchins L, Craig M, Fojo AT, Wright JJ, Bates SE. Phase 2 trial of romidepsin in patients with peripheral T-cell lymphoma. *Blood* 2011, 117, 5827-5834.

[52] McDermott J, Jimeno A. Belinostat for the treatment of peripheral T-cell lymphomas. *Drugs Today (Barc)* 2014, 50, 337-345.

[53] Coiffier B, Federico M, Caballero D, Dearden C, Morschhauser F, Jäger U, Trümper L, Zucca E, Gomes da Silva M, Pettengell R, Weidmann E, d'Amore F, Tilly H, Zinzani PL. Therapeutic options in relapsed or refractory peripheral T-cell lymphoma. *Cancer Treat. Rev.* 2014, 40, 1080-1088.

[54] Poole RM. Belinostat: first global approval. *Drugs* 2014, 74, 1543-1554.

[55] Reimer P, Chawla S. Long-term complete remission with belinostat in a patient with chemotherapy refractory peripheral T-cell lymphoma. *J. Hematol. Oncol.* 2013, 6, 69.

[56] Guenova E, Hoetzenecker W, Rozati S, Levesque MP, Dummer R, Cozzio A. Novel therapies for cutaneous T-cell lymphoma: what does the future hold? *Expert Opin. Investig. Drugs* 2014, 23, 457-467.

[57] Piekarz RL, Frye R, Turner M, Wright JJ, Allen SL, Kirschbaum MH, Zain J, Prince HM, Leonard JP, Geskin LJ, Reeder C, Joske D, Figg

WD, Gardner ER, Steinberg SM, Jaffe ES, Stetler-Stevenson M, Lade S, Fojo AT, Bates SE. Phase II multi-institutional trial of the histone deacetylase inhibitor romidepsin as monotherapy for patients with cutaneous T-cell lymphoma. J. Clin. Oncol. 2009, 27, 5410-5417.

[58] Olsen EA, Kim YH, Kuzel TM, Pacheco TR, Foss FM, Parker S, Frankel SR, Chen C, Ricker JL, Arduino JM, Duvic M. Phase IIb multicenter trial of vorinostat in patients with persistent, progressive, or treatment refractory cutaneous T-cell lymphoma. *J. Clin. Oncol.* 2007, 25, 3109-3115.

[59] Ellis L, Pan Y, Smyth GK, George DJ, McCormack C, Williams-Truax R, Mita M, Beck J, Burris H, Ryan G, Atadja P, Butterfoss D, Dugan M, Culver K, Johnstone RW, Prince HM. Histone deacetylase inhibitor panobinostat induces clinical responses with associated alterations in gene expression profiles in cutaneous T-cell lymphoma. *Clin. Cancer Res.* 2008, 14, 4500-4510.

[60] Whittaker SJ, Demierre MF, Kim EJ, Rook AH, Lerner A, Duvic M, Scarisbrick J, Reddy S, Robak T, Becker JC, Samtsov A, McCulloch W, Kim YH. Final results from a multicenter, international, pivotal study of romidepsin in refractory cutaneous T-cell lymphoma. *J. Clin. Oncol.* 2010, 28, 4485-4491.

[61] Lyseng-Williamson KA, Yang LP. Romidepsin: a guide to its clinical use in cutaneous T-cell lymphoma. *Am. J. Clin. Dermatol.* 2012, 13, 67-71.

[62] McGraw AL. Romidepsin for the treatment of T-cell lymphomas. *Am. J. Health Syst. Pharm.* 2013, 70, 1115-1122.

[63] Kim YH, Demierre MF, Kim EJ, Lerner A, Rook AH, Duvic M, Robak T, Samtsov A, McCulloch W, Chen SC, Waksman J, Nichols J, Whittaker S. Clinically meaningful reduction in pruritus in patients with cutaneous T-cell lymphoma treated with romidepsin. *Leuk. Lymphoma* 2013, 54, 284-289.

[64] Moskowitz AJ. Novel agents in Hodgkin lymphoma. *Clin. Oncol. Rep.* 2012, 14, 419-423.

[65] Bolden JE, Peart MJ, Johnstone RW. Anticancer activities of histone deacetylase inhibitors. *Nat. Rev. Drug Discov.* 2006, 5, 769–784.

[66] Cotto M, Cabanillas F, Tirado M, et al. Epigenetic therapy of lymphoma using histone deacetylase inhibitors. *Clin. Transl. Oncol.* 2010, 12, 401–409.

[67] Lane AA, Chabner BA. Histone deacetylase inhibitors in cancer therapy. *J. Clin. Oncol.* 2009, 27, 5459–5468.

[68] Younes A. Novel treatment strategies for patients with relapsed classical Hodgkin lymphoma. *Hematology Am. Soc. Hematol. Educ. Program* 2009, 2009, 507–519.

[69] Ushmorov A, Leithauser F, Sakk O, et al. Epigenetic processes play a major role in B-cell-specific gene silencing in classical Hodgkin lymphoma. *Blood* 2006, 107, 2493–2500.

[70] Ramchandren R. Advances in the Treatment of Relapsed or Refractory Hodgkin's Lymphoma. *Oncologist* 2012, 17, 367-376.

[71] Oki Y, Copeland A, Younes A. Clinical development of panobinostat in classical Hodgkin's lymphoma. *Expert Rev. Hematol.* 2011, 4, 245-252.

[72] Blum KA. Upcoming diagnostic and therapeutic developments in classical Hodgkin's lymphoma. *Hematology Am. Soc. Hematol. Educ. Program* 2010, 2010, 93–100.

[73] Younes A, Oki Y, Bociek RG, Kuruvilla J, Fanale M, Neelapu S, Copeland A, Buglio D, Galal A, Besterman J, Li Z, Drouin M, Patterson T, Ward MR, Paulus JK, Ji Y, Medeiros LJ, Martell RE. Mocetinostat for relapsed classical Hodgkin's lymphoma: an open-label, single-arm, phase 2 trial. *Lancet Oncol.* 2011, 12, 1222-1228.

[74] Oki Y, Buglio D, Fanale M, Fayad L, Copeland A, Romaguera J, Kwak LW, Pro B, de Castro Faria S, Neelapu S, Fowler N, Hagemeister F, Zhang J, Zhou S, Feng L, Younes A. Phase I study of panobinostat plus everolimus in patients with relapsed or refractory lymphoma. *Clin. Cancer Res.* 2013, 19, 6882-6890.

[75] Provencio M, Sánchez A, Sánchez-Beato M. New drugs and targeted treatments in Hodgkin's lymphoma. *Cancer Treat. Rev*. 2014, 40, 457-464.

[76] von Tresckow B, Diehl V. An update on emerging drugs for Hodgkin lymphoma. *Expert Opin. Emerg. Drugs* 2014, 19, 215-224.

[77] Oki Y, Buglio D, Zhang J, Ying Y, Zhou S, Sureda A, Ben-Yehuda D, Zinzani PL, Prince HM, Harrison SJ, Kirschbaum M, Johnston PB, Shen A, von Tresckow B, Younes A. Immune regulatory effects of panobinostat in patients with Hodgkin lymphoma through modulation of serum cytokine levels and T-cell PD1 expression. *Blood Cancer J.* 2014, 4, e236.

[78] Buglio D, Khaskhely NM, Voo KS, Martinez-Valdez H, Liu YJ, Younes A. HDAC11 plays an essential role in regulating OX40 ligand expression in Hodgkin lymphoma. *Blood* 2011, 117, 2910–2917.

[79] Klein JM, Henke A, Sauer M, Bessler M, Reiners KS, Engert A, et al. The histone deacetylase inhibitor LBH589 (panobinostat) modulates the

crosstalk of lymphocytes with Hodgkin lymphoma cell lines. *PloS One* 2013, 8, e79502.

[80] Younes A, Sureda A, Ben-Yehuda D, Zinzani PL, Ong TC, Prince HM, et al. Panobinostat in patients with relapsed/refractory Hodgkin's lymphoma after autologous stem-cell transplantation: results of a phase II study. *J. Clin. Oncol.* 2012, 30, 2197–2203.

[81] Harrison SJ, Hsu AK, Neeson P, Younes A, Sureda A, Engert A, et al. Early thymus and activation-regulated chemokine (TARC) reduction and response following panobinostat treatment in patients with relapsed/refractory Hodgkin lymphoma following autologous stem cell transplant. *Leuk. Lymphoma* 2014, 55, 1053–1060.

[82] Advani AS, Gibson SE, Douglas E, Jin T, Zhao X, Kalaycio M, Copelan E, Sobecks R, Sekeres M, Sungren S, Hsi ED. Histone H4 acetylation by immunohistochemistry and prognosis in newly diagnosed adult acute lymphoblastic leukemia (ALL) patients. *BMC Cancer* 2010, 10, 387.

[83] Tsapis M, Lieb M, Manzo F, Shankaranarayanan P, Herbrecht R, Lutz P, Gronemeyer H. HDAC inhibitors induce apoptosis in glucocorticoid-resistant acute lymphatic leukemia cells despite a switch from the extrinsic to the intrinsic death pathway. *Int. J. Biochem. Cell Biol.* 2007, 39, 1500-1509.

[84] Lo Nigro L. Biology of childhood acute lymphoblastic leukemia. *J. Pediatr. Hematol. Oncol.* 2013, 35, 245-252.

[85] Stams WA, den Boer ML, Beverloo HB, Kazemier KM, van Wering ER, Janka-Schaub GE, Pieters R. Effect of the histone deacetylase inhibitor depsipeptide on B-cell differentiation in both TEL-AML1-positive and negative childhood acute lymphoblastic leukemia. *Haematologica* 2005, 90, 1697-1699.

[86] Haggarty SJ, Koeller KM, Wong JC, Grozinger CM, Schreiber SL. Domain-selective small-molecule inhibitor of histone deacetylase 6 (HDAC6)-mediated tubulin deacetylation. *Proc. Natl. Acad. Sci. U S A.* 2003, 100, 4389-4394.

[87] Aldana-Masangkay GI, Rodriguez-Gonzalez A, Lin T, Ikeda AK, Hsieh YT, Kim YM, Lomenick B, Okemoto K, Landaw EM, Wang D, Mazitschek R, Bradner JE, Sakamoto KM. Tubacin suppresses proliferation and induces apoptosis of acute lymphoblastic leukemia cells. *Leuk. Lymphoma* 2011, 52, 1544-1555.

[88] Eklund EA, Platanias LC. Inhibition of histone deacetylase 6 as a therapeutic strategy for acute lymphocytic leukemia. *Leuk. Lymphoma* 2011, 52, 1421-1422.

[89] Wang JC, Kafeel MI, Avezbakiyev B, Chen C, Sun Y, Rathnasabapathy C, Kalavar M, He Z, Burton J, Lichter S. Histone deacetylase in chronic lymphocytic leukemia. *Oncology* 2011, 81, 325-329.

[90] Herishanu Y, Katz BZ, Lipsky A, Wiestner A. Biology of chronic lymphocytic leukemia in different microenvironments. Clinical and therapeutic implications. *Hematol. Oncol. Clin. N. Amer.* 2013, 27, 173-206.

[91] Amin S, Walsh M, Wilson C, Parker AE, Oscier D, Willmore E, Mann D, Mann J. Cross-talk between DNA methylation and active histone modifications regulates aberrant expression of ZAP70 in CLL. *J. Cell. Mol. Med.* 2012, 16, 2074-2084.

[92] Pérez-Perarnau A, Coll-Mulet L, Rubio-Patiño C, Iglesias-Serret D, Cosialls AM, González-Gironès DM, de Frias M, de Sevilla AF, de la Banda E, Pons G, Gil J. Analysis of apoptosis regulatory genes altered by histone deacetylase inhibitors in chronic lymphocytic leukemia cells. *Epigenetics* 2011, 6, 1228-1235.

[93] El-Khoury V, Moussay E, Janji B, Palissot V, Aouali N, Brons NH, Van Moer K, Pierson S, Van Dyck E, Berchem G. The histone deacetylase inhibitor MGCD0103 induces apoptosis in B-cell chronic lymphocytic leukemia cells through a mitochondria-mediated caspase activation cascade. *Mol. Cancer Ther.* 2010, 9, 1349-1360.

[94] El-Khoury V, Pierson S, Szwarcbart E, Brons NH, Roland O, Cherrier-De Wilde S, Plawny L, Van Dyck E, Berchem G. Disruption of autophagy by the histone deacetylase inhibitor MGCD0103 and its therapeutic implication in B-cell chronic lymphocytic leukemia. *Leukemia* 2014, 28, 1636-1646.

[95] Lavelle D, Chen YH, Hankewych M, DeSimone J. Histone deacetylase inhibitors increase p21(WAF1) and induce apoptosis of human myeloma cell lines independent of decreased IL-6 receptor expression. *Am. J. Hematol.* 2001, 68, 170–178.

[96] Mitsiades N, Mitsiades CS, Richardson PG, McMullan C, Poulaki V, Fanourakis G, Schlossman R, Chauhan D, Munshi NC, Hideshima T, Richon VM, Marks PA, Anderson KC. Molecular sequelae of histone deacetylase inhibition in human malignant B cells. *Blood* 2003, 101, 4055–4062.

[97] Khan SB, Maududi T, Barton K, Ayers J, Alkan S. Analysis of histone deacetylase inhibitor, depsipeptide (FR901228), effect on multiple myeloma. *Br. J. Haematol.* 2004, 125, 156–161.

[98] Feng R, Ma H, Hassig CA, Payne JE, Smith ND, Mapara MY, Hager JH, Lentzsch S. KD5170, a novel mercaptoketone-based histone deacetylase inhibitor, exerts antimyeloma effects by DNA damage and mitochondrial signaling. *Mol. Cancer Ther.* 2008, 7, 1494–1505.

[99] Neri P, Tagliaferri P, Di Martino MT, Calimeri T, Amodio N, Bulotta A, Ventura M, Eramo PO, Viscomi C, Arbitrio M, Rossi M, Caraglia M, Munshi NC, Anderson KC, Tassone P. *In vivo* anti-myeloma activity and modulation of gene expression profile induced by valproic acid, a histone deacetylase inhibitor. *Br. J. Haematol.* 2008, 143, 520–531.

[100] Neri P, Bahlis NJ, Lonial S. Panobinostat for the treatment of multiple myeloma. *Expert Opin. Investig. Drugs* 2012, 21, 733–747.

[101] Rao R, Nalluri S, Kolhe R, Yang Y, Fiskus W, Chen J, Ha K, Buckley KM, Balusu R, Coothankandaswamy V, Joshi A, Atadja P, Bhalla KN. Treatment with panobinostat induces glucose-regulated protein 78 acetylation and endoplasmic reticulum stress in breast cancer cells. *Mol. Cancer Ther.* 2010, 9, 942–952.

[102] Kahali S, Sarcar B, Chinnaiyan P. The emerging role of histone deacetylases (HDACs) in UPR regulation. *Methods Enzymol.* 2011, 490, 159–174.

[103] Kahali S, Sarcar B, Prabhu A, Seto E, Chinnaiyan P. Class I histone deacetylases localize to the endoplasmic reticulum and modulate the unfolded protein response. *FASEB J.* 2012, 26, 2437–2445.

[104] Hideshima T, Anderson KC. Histone deacetylase inhibitors in the treatment for multiple myeloma. *Int. J. Hematol.* 2013, 97, 324–332.

[105] Richardson P, Mitsiades C, Colson K, Reilly E, McBride L, Chiao J, Sun L, Ricker J, Rizvi S, Oerth C, Atkins B, Fearen I, Anderson K, Siegel D. Phase I trial of oral vorinostat (suberoylanilide hydroxamic acid, SAHA) in patients with advanced multiple myeloma. *Leuk. Lymphoma* 2008, 49, 502–507.

[106] Niesvizky R, Ely S, Mark T, Aggarwal S, Gabrilove JL, Wright JJ, Chen-Kiang S, Sparano JA. Phase 2 trial of the histone deacetylase inhibitor romidepsin for the treatment of refractory multiple myeloma. *Cancer* 2011, 117, 336–342.

[107] Badros A, Burger AM, Philip S, Niesvizky R, Kolla SS, Goloubeva O, Harris C, Zwiebel J, Wright JJ, Espinoza-Delgado I, Baer MR, Holleran JL, Egorin MJ, Grant S. Phase I study of vorinostat in combination with bortezomib for relapsed and refractory multiple myeloma. *Clin. Cancer Res.* 2009, 15, 5250–5257.

[108] Harrison SJ, Quach H, Link E, Seymour JF, Ritchie DS, Ruell S, Dean J, Januszewicz H, Johnstone R, Neeson P, Dickinson M, Nichols J, Prince HM. A high rate of durable responses with romidepsin, bortezomib, and dexamethasone in relapsed or refractory multiple myeloma. *Blood* 2011, 118, 6274–6283.

[109] Moreaux J, Reme T, Leonard W, Veyrune JL, Requirand G, Goldschmidt H, Hose D, Klein B. Development of gene expression-based score to predict sensitivity of multiple myeloma cells to DNA methylation inhibitors. *Mol. Cancer Ther.* 2012, 11, 2685–2692.

[110] Ocio EM, Richardson PG, Rajkumar SV, Palumbo A, Mateos MV, Orlowski R, Kumar S, Usmani S, Roodman D, Niesvizky R, Einsele H, Anderson KC, Dimopoulos MA, Avet-Loiseau H, Mellqvist UH, Turesson I, Merlini G, Schots R, McCarthy P, Bergsagel L, Chim CS, Lahuerta JJ, Shah J, Reiman A, Mikhael J, Zweegman S, Lonial S, Comenzo R, Chng WJ, Moreau P, Sonneveld P, Ludwig H, Durie BG, Miguel JF. New drugs and novel mechanisms of action in multiple myeloma in 2013: a report from the International Myeloma Working Group (IMWG). *Leukemia* 2014, 28, 525-542.

[111] Jagannath S, Dimopoulos MA, Lonial S. Combined proteasome and histone deacetylase inhibition: A promising synergy for patients with relapsed/refractory multiple myeloma. *Leuk. Res* 2010, 34, 1111-1118.

[112] Hideshima T, Richardson PG, Anderson KC. Mechanism of action of proteasome inhibitors and deacetylase inhibitors and the biological basis of synergy in multiple myeloma. *Mol. Cancer Ther.* 2011, 10, 2034-2042.

[113] Santo L, Hideshima T, Kung AL, Tseng JC, Tamang D, Yang M, Jarpe M, van Duzer JH, Mazitschek R, Ogier WC, Cirstea D, Rodig S, Eda H, Scullen T, Canavese M, Bradner J, Anderson KC, Jones SS, Raje N. Preclinical activity, pharmacodynamic, and pharmacokinetic properties of a selective HDAC6 inhibitor, ACY-1215, in combination with bortezomib in multiple myeloma. *Blood* 2012, 119, 2579-2589.

[114] Ghobrial IM, Campigotto F, Murphy TJ, Boswell EN, Banwait R, Azab F, Chuma S, Kunsman J, Donovan A, Masood F, Warren D, Rodig S, Anderson KC, Richardson PG, Weller E, Matous J. Results of a phase 2 trial of the single-agent histone deacetylase inhibitor panobinostat in patients with relapsed/refractory Waldenström macroglobulinemia. *Blood* 2013, 121, 1296-1303.

[115] Dai Y, Rahmani M, Dent P, Grant S. Blockade of Histone Deacetylase Inhibitor-Induced RelA/p65 Acetylation and NF-{kappa}B Activation

Potentiates Apoptosis in Leukemia Cells through a Process Mediated by Oxidative Damage, XIAP Downregulation, and c-Jun N-Terminal Kinase 1 Activation. *Mol. Cell. Biol.* 2005, 25, 5429–5444.

[116] Grant S. Targeting Waldenstrom macroglobulinemia with histone deacetylase inhibitors. *Leuk. Lymphoma* 2011, 52, 1623-1625.

[117] Sun JY, Tseng H, Xu L, Hunter Z, Ciccarelli B, Fulciniti M, Zhu B, Maghsoudi K, Yang G, Gong P, Zhou Y, Liu X, Munshi NC, Patterson CJ, Treon SP. Vorinostat induced cellular stress disrupts the p38 mitogen activated protein kinase and extracellular signal regulated kinase pathways leading to apoptosis in Waldenström macroglobulinemia cells. *Leuk. Lymphoma* 2011, 52, 1777-1786.

[118] Peiffer L, Poll-Wolbeck SJ, Flamme H, Gehrke I, Hallek M, Kreuzer KA. Trichostatin A effectively induces apoptosis in chronic lymphocytic leukemia via inhibition of Wnt signaling and histone deacetylation. *J. Cancer Res. Clin. Oncol.* 2014, 140, 1283-1293.

[119] Gandhirajan RK, Poll-Wolbeck SJ, Gehrke I, Kreuzer KA. Wnt/β-catenin/LEF-1 signaling in chronic lymphocytic leukemia (CLL): a target for current and potential therapeutic options. *Curr. Cancer Drug Targets* 2010, 10, 716-727.

[120] Thanendrarajan S, Kim Y, Schmidt-Wolf IG. Understanding and targeting the Wnt/β-catenin signaling pathway in chronic leukemia. *Leuk. Res. Treatment* 2011, 2011, 329572.

[121] Jordaan G, Liao V, Sharma S. E-cadherin gene re-expression in chronic lymphocytic leukemia cells by HDAC inhibitors. *BMC Cancer* 2013, 13, 88.

[122] Fuchs O. Promising activity of mammalian target of rapamycin inhibitors in hematologic malignancies therapy. *Curr. Signal Transduction Therapy* 2011, 6, 44-54.

[123] Simmons JK, Patel J, Michalowski A, Zhang S, Wei BR, Sullivan P, Gamache B, Felsenstein K, Kuehl WM, Simpson RM, Zingone A, Landgren O, Mock BA. TORC1 and class I HDAC inhibitors synergize to suppress mature B cell neoplasms. *Mol. Oncol.* 2014, 8, 261-272.

[124] Fuchs O. Targeting of NF-κB signaling pathway, other signaling pathways and epigenetics in therapy of multiple myeloma. *Cardiovasc. Hematol. Disorders Drug Targets* 2013, 13, 16-34.

[125] Orlowski RZ. Novel agents for multiple myeloma to overcome resistance in phase III clinical trials. *Semin. Oncol.* 2013, 40, 634-651.

In: Histone Deacetylase Inhibitors (HDIs)
Editor: Beverly D. Carson ISBN: 978-1-63463-835-7

Chapter 3

HISTONE DEACETYLASE INHIBITORS IN THE TREATMENT OF MYELOID MALIGNANCIES

Ota Fuchs[1]
Institute of Hematology and Blood Transfusion
Prague, Czech Republic

ABSTRACT

The results of current treatment for patients with acute myeloid leukemia (AML) remain poor and there is a need for innovative strategies. Epigenetic modulation became a promising approach. A number of clinical trials have studied the safety and clinical activity of histone deacetylase (HDAC) inhibitors (HDACIs) in AML and myelodysplastic syndrome (MDS). All classes of HDACIs were used: hydroxamic acids (vorinostat and panobinostat); cyclic peptide (romidepsin); benzamides (mocetinostat and entinostat); fatty acids (valproic acid). The conclusion of these studies with HDACI as a single agent was that the best use of these compounds would be in combination with other antileukemia agents. Aberrant promoter DNA hypermethylation and histone deacetylation are reversible processes implicated in myeloid leukemogenesis. A phase 1 trial looking at romidepsin and the hypomethylating agent azacitidine for AML (ROMAZA) was opened (2013-2015) in England. This trial is for patients with newly diagnosed relapsed or refractory AML who can't have

[1] Corresponding author: Ota Fuchs, PhD, Tel: 420 221977512; Fax: 420 221977370, E-mail: Ota.Fuchs@uhkt.cz.

standard chemotherapy treatment. In the US the similar phase 1 trial with AR-142, the novel orally bioavailable HDACI, and decitabine is provided (2013-2015). The wild-type p53 is required for induction of cell death by azacitidine in combination with romidepsin or panobinostat. Increasing anti-leukemic activity of decitabine via AR-42-induced upregulation of miR-29b and downregulation of known miR-29b targets (transcription factor SP1, DNA methyltransferases DNMT1, DNMT3A and DNMT3B) is a novel epigenetic targeting approach in AML. The combination of vorinostat with the DNA topoisomerase inhibitor idarubicin had synergistic antileukemia effect. Combinations of vorinostat with cytosine arabinoside (cytarabine) and another DNA topoisomerase inhibitor etoposide had also potent antileukemia activity. Vorinostat induces reactive oxygen species (ROS) that results in translocation of transcription factor NRF2 (nuclear factor-erythroid-2-related factor 2) from the cytoplasm to nucleus. This in turn results in the activation of expression of anti-oxidant genes involved in overcoming of ROS pathway. Valproic acid (VPA) monotherapy inhibits the proliferation of leukemic cells regardless of the expression of p-glycoprotein and multidrug resistance associated protein 1. VPA has been more frequently studied in the combinations, specifically with all- trans retinoic acid (ATRA). VPA was also combined with both ATRA and azacitidine. Phase 1 and 2 trials with panobinostat and phase 2 study of vorinostat in patients with primary myelofibrosis and post-polycythemia vera/essential thrombocythemia myelofibrosis were associated with clinical improvement with 100% reduction palpable splenomegaly and with improvement in the degree of anemia. Gene expression profiling and epigenome studies during treatment with HDACIs are ongoing in an attempt to clarify particular patterns of gene and epigenome deregulation that is necessary for a better understanding of clinical and biochemical effects of HDACIs.

Keywords: Acetylation, acute myeloid leukemia, apoptosis, cell cycle, chronic myeloid leukemia, HDAC inhibitors, histone deacetylates, myelodysplastic syndrome, primary myelofibrosis

INTRODUCTION

Epigenetics is the study of herritable changes in gene expression. These changes are not due to modifications in the DNA sequence. Epigenetic changes include DNA methylation, histone modifications and the action of small non-coding RNAs (ncRNA) that can regulate gene expression. Post-translational modifications that occur on certain amino acid residues of the tails of histone proteins modify chromatin structure and thereby alter gene expression. Among the histone covalent modifications histone acetylation is the most well understood. The enzyme histone acetyl transferase (HAT) acetylates lysine residues at the N terminus of histone protein and histone deacetylase (HDAC) removes acetyl groups from histone. These chemical modifications on the histones form the basis for "histone code" [1-5]. Such histone modifications may be associated with gene expression or gene silencing. For example, acetylation of lysine 9 on histone 3 is associated with gene activation whereas acetylation of lysine 16 on histone 4 leads to gene repression. HDAC inhibitors (HDACIs) impact chromatin conformation by altering the pattern of acetylation of lysine residues in nucleosomal histones. HDACIs promote acetylation of histone which neutralizes the positive charge of the histone tails and reduces the affinity of histone for the negatively charged DNA. This loosens the structure of the chromatin to an open configuration which enables the transcriptional machinery to access the DNA and enhance gene transcription. Secondly, HDACIs promote acetylation of non-histone protein substrates, such as DNA-binding proteins, transcription factors, signal-transduction molecules, DNA-repair proteins, and chaperone proteins. These modifications of the non-histone proteins can affect many vital regulatory processes, including gene expression, mRNA stability, protein activity, and protein stability. HDACIs have also other functions including effect on cell cycle, antiangiogenic effect, inhibition of DNA repair, induction of reactive oxygen species, inhibition of protein chaperone, disruption of aggresome formation, effect on cell cycle, effect on immune cells, induction of apoptosis, alteration of death receptor pathways, and alterations of NF-κB pathway [5-16]. Via autophagy suppression, HDACIs deprive cells of an essential pro-survival mechanism, which translates into an attractive strategy to specifically target cancer cells [17].

HDACIs in Myelodysplastic Syndrome Therapy

Myelodysplastic syndromes (MDS) are a diverse group of clonal hematopoietic stem cell disorders manifested by ineffective production of blood cells with varying need for transfusions, risk of infection, and risk of transformation to AML. Epigenetic changes, such as DNA methylation, histone acetylation, and RNA interference, alter gene expression, impacting disease biology and play important role in the pathogenesis of MDS. Hypermethylation of CpG islands in the promoter of key genes involved in cell cycle regulation, apoptosis, tumor suppression, and response to chemotherapy, and the consequent silencing of their expression is well documented in MDS. Hypermethylated DNA sequences of key cellular machinery provide an attractive therapeutic target for the treatment of MDS. Histone modification, another route of gene expression control, is also involved in the biopathologic process of MDS. DNA methylation and histone modification not only regulate the expression of protein-encoding genes but also microRNAs (miRs), such as let-7a, miR-9, miR-34a, miR-124, miR-137, miR-148 and miR-203. Hypomethylating (demethylating) agents are cytidine analogues that establish an irreversible covalent bond with DNA methyltransferases (DNMTs) after DNA incorporation. DNMT inhibitors are now approved for clinical use to treat MDS. 5-Aza-cytidine (Vidaza) and 5-aza-2'-deoxycytidine (5-azaCdR; decitabine) have become the standard in the treatment of patients with higher-risk MDS, in particular older individuals, where intensive chemotherapy and allogeneic stem cell transplantation are not possible. Drugs that alter histone modification are also available and being studied in MDS.

The role of chromatin remodeling in carcinogenesis was studied with the help of inhibitors of HDACs (HDACIs). HDACIs induce the hyperacetylation of nucleosomal histones in cells resulting in the expression of aberrantly repressed genes (e.g., tumor suppressor genes) that produce growth arrest, terminal differentiation, and/or apoptosis in carcinoma cells, depending on the HDACI and dose used, and the cell type [18-21]. The inappropriate recruitment of HDACs provides at least one mechanism by which oncogenes could alter gene expression in favor of excessive proliferation. Thus, orally active HDACIs with low toxicity towards normal cells and tissues, which would effectively inhibit tumor growth are needed for epigenetic anticancer therapy. In October 2006, the US Food and Drug Administration (FDA) approved the first drug of this new class, vorinostat (SAHA, Zolinza) for treatment of cutaneous T-cell lymphoma. Several further HDIs (romidepsin, belinostat, sodium phenylbutyrate, valproic acid, entinostat, and mocetinostat) are in clinical trials. HDACIs have shown significant activity against a variety of hematological and solid tumors at doses that are well tolerated by patients, both in monotherapy as well as in combination therapy with other drugs. Combined DNA methyltransferase and histone deacetylase inhibition are used in experiments *in vitro* but also in clinical trials in MDS patients [8, 22-28].

In a preclinical study, epigenetically silenced tumor suppressor genes, *MLH1, TIMP3,CDKN2A,* and *CDKN2B*, were reexpressed following combination treatment with decitabine and the HDACI trichostatin A [22].

Clinical data of HDACIs alone or in combination with azacitidine are described below and are summarized in the recent paper [29].

Vorinostat (suberoylanilide hydroxamic acid; SAHA) was tested in single-agent phase 1 study in 41 patients with hematologic malignancies including 31 AML, 3 MDS, 2 acute lymphoblastic leukemia (ALL), and 1 chronic myelomonocytic leukemia (CMML) [30]. Responses were observed in 7 of 41 enrolled patients, including 2 complete response (CR) and 2 CR with incomplete blood count recovery, all in patients with AML.

Vorinostat in combination with the DNA topoisomerase inhibitor idarubicin and ara-C (cytarabine) was nevaluated in a phase 2 study of 75 patients with AML or high-risk MDS. Median age was 52 years (range, 19 to 65 years), 29 patients (39%) were cytogenetically normal, and 11 (15%) had FLT-3 internal tandem duplication (ITD). No excess vorinostat-related toxicity was observed. Induction mortality was 4%. EFS was 47 weeks (range, 3 to 134 weeks), and overall survival was 82 weeks (range, 3 to 134 weeks). Overall response rate (ORR) was 85%, including 76% CR and 9% in CR with incomplete platelet recovery. ORR was 93% in diploid patients and 100% in FLT-3 ITD patients. Levels of the nuclear factor erythroid 2-related factor (NRF2) and cytochrome b-245, beta subunit (CYBB) were associated with longer survival. NRF2 is a transcription factor that functions as the key controller of the redox homeostatic gene regulatory network. CYBB (also known as p91-phox) is one part (subunit) of a group of proteins that forms an enzyme complex called NADPH oxidase, which plays an essential role in the immune system. The combination of vorinostat with idarubicin and cytarabine is safe and active in AML. The most common grade 1/2 adverse events (AEs) were nausea/vomiting (53%), diarrhea (35%), skin toxicities (33%) and other GI toxicities (24%). Common grade 3/4 AEs included diarrhea (36%) and other *gastrointestinal* (GI) toxicities (15%).

In phase 1 study, depsipeptide (romidepsin) was administered to MDS or AML patients at a dose of 18 mg/m^2 i.v. on days 1 and 5 every 3 weeks [32]. Toxicities and clinical activity were monitored and pharmacokinetic and pharmacodynamic studies were done. Twelve patients (nine with AML, three with MDS) received one to five cycles of depsipeptide. The most common grade 3/4 toxicities were febrile neutropenia/infection (5 patients), neutropenia/thrombocytopenia (9 patients), nausea (9 patients), and asymptomatic hypophosphatemia (3 patients). No clinically significant cardiac toxicity was observed. The best response of 11 assessed patients was one complete remission in a patient with AML, stable disease in six patients, and progression of disease in four patients. Exploratory laboratory studies showed modest but rapid increases in apoptosis and changes in myeloid maturation marker expression. Histone H3 and H4 acetylation levels were evaluated in five patients; no consistent changes were observed. Depsipeptide therapy can be administered with acceptable short-term toxicity. However, gastrointestinal symptoms and fatigue seem to be treatment-limiting after multiple cycles. Depsipeptide monotherapy has limited clinical activity in unselected AML/MDS patients [32].

Valproic acid (VPA) has been used as an anticonvulsant for decades. Recently, it was demonstrated that VPA also acts as a HDACI and induces differentiation and apoptosis in a variety of malignant cells in vitro [33]. VPA has been shown to inhibit HDAC activity and to synergize with all-trans retinoic acid (ATRA) in the differentiation induction of AML blasts in vitro. Therefore, 18 patients with MDS and AML secondary to MDS (sAML/MDS) was treated with VPA monotherapy (serum concentrations 346-693 μM [50-100 μg/mL]) [34, 35]. Five patients received VPA and ATRA (80 mg/m^2)/d, days 1-7, every other week). Response according to international working group (IWG) criteria was observed in 8 patients (44%) on VPA monotherapy, including 1 partial remission. Median response duration was 4 months (range, 3-9 months). Four of 5 patients relapsing were treated with VPA + ATRA, 2 of them responded again. Among 5 patients receiving VPA + ATRA from the start, none responded according to IWG criteria, but 1 patient with sAML/MDS achieved a marked reduction in peripheral and marrow blasts. Thus, VPA is of therapeutic benefit for patients with MDS, and ATRA may be effective when added later [34, 35]. Follow-up data were reported on 75 patients [36]. Of these, 66 were started on VPA monotherapy, with later addition of ATRA in patients who did not respond or relapsed. Nine patients were treated with VPA + ATRA from the start. Median treatment duration was 4 months for VPA and 2 months for ATRA. Hematological improvement, according to international working group criteria for MDS, was observed in 18 patients (24%). Median response duration was 4 months. ATRA exerted no additional effect in patients receiving the combination from the start or benefited primary VPA nonresponders. However, of 10 VPA responders who relapsed, 4 achieved a second response after addition of ATRA. Response rates were strongly dependent on disease type according to WHO classification. The response rate of 52% in MDS patients with a normal blast count (refractory sideroblastic anemia, refractory cytopenia with multilineage dysplasia, and refractory sideroblastic cytopenia with multilineage dysplasia) was found. The response rate was 6% in refractory anemia with excess blasts

(I + II), 16% in AML, and 0% in chronic myelomonocytic leukemia. Bone marrow blast count was the only variable that predicted responses. It was concluded that VPA is clinically useful in low-risk MDS [36]. For patients with high-risk MDS, VPA may be combined with chemotherapy or demethylating drugs. If patients relapse after an initial response to VPA, ATRA has the potential to induce a prolonged second response.

Two phase 1/2 studies evaluated the combination of decitabine (5-aza-2'-deoxycytidine, DAC) with VPA. The first used DAC 15 mg/m^2/day for 10 days with a dose escalation of VPA from 20 to 50 mg/kg/day for 10 days in patients with high grade MDS or AML [24]. Fifty four patients of median age 60 (range 5–80 years) were enrolled, 48 patients had AML and 6 had MDS, 11 patients were previously untreated. Twelve patients responded to therapy; 10 developed a CR and 2 a CR with incomplete platelet recovery. Median responses were seen after 2 months (range 29–130 days) and responders survived a median of 15.3 (range 4.6–20.2+) months vs. 4.9 (0.6–17.8+) months in non-responders [24]. Responders were more likely to have been randomized to a higher dose of valproic acid. Although changes in methylation (both gene specific events, including *p15INK4B*, and genome wide methylation, by LINE-1 /Long Interspersed Element-1/ pyrosequencing) and gene expression were analyzed in the patients on this study no correlations with response were observed [24]. Bisulfite conversion and PCR pyrosequencing assay can measure LINE-1methylation and may be useful in clinical and research. All patients experienced a decrease in genome wide methylation which correlated with DAC exposure. In a second study DAC 20 mg/m^2/day for 10 days intravenously, responses were also encouraging with an overall response rate of 44% in 11 of 25 enrolled patients [37]. This trial enrolled 25 AML patients, in whom the median age was 70 years; 12 patients were untreated and 13 had relapsed disease. In this group of slightly older patients, encephalopathy was the principal toxicity and this was dose limiting at 20–25 mg/kg/day. In an intent-to-treat analysis, the response rate was 52% (13). CR was observed in 8 patients and PR in 4. Responses appeared similar for patients who received DAC alone and for those who received valproic acid in addition. In this study, re-expression of estrogen receptor (ER) was statistically significantly associated with clinical response ($p = 0.05$), however although the investigators also demonstrated ER promoter demethylation, global DNA hypomethylation, depletion of DNA methyltransferase enzyme, and histone hyperacetylation, these markers did not correlate with response [37].

5-azacytidine (AZA) has become standard treatment for patients with higher-risk MDS. Response rate is about 50% and response duration is limited. HDACIs are attractive partners for epigenetic combination therapy. Twenty four patients were treated with AZA (100 mg/m^2, 5 days) plus VPA; continuous dosing, serum level 80-110 μg/ml) [38]. According to WHO classification, 5 patients had MDS, 2 had MDS/MPD, and 17 had AML. Seven patients (29%) had previously received intensive chemotherapy, and five had previous HDACI treatment. Common grade 3/4 AEs included neutropenic fever (12%) and pneumonia (10%). The overall response rate was 37% in the entire cohort but significantly higher (57%) in previously untreated patients, especially those with MDS (64%). Seven (29%) patients achieved CR (29%) and two PR (8%), respectively. Hematological CR was accompanied by complete cytogenetic remission according to conventional cytogenetics in all evaluable cases. Some patients also showed complete remission according to FISH on bone marrow mononuclear cells and CD34$^+$ peripheral blood cells, as well as by follow-up of somatic mitochondrial DNA mutations. Four additional patients achieved at least marrow remissions. Factors influencing response were AML (vs. MDS), marrow blast count, pretreatment, transfusion dependency, concomitant medication with hydroxyurea, and valproic acid (VPA) serum level. This trial is the first to assess the combination of AZA plus VPA without additional ATRA. A comparatively good CR rate, relatively short time to response, and the influence of VPA serum levels on response suggest that VPA provided substantial additional benefit [38]. However, the importance of HDACIs in epigenetic combination therapy can only be proven by randomized trials.

Pracinostat (SB 939) is a HDACI with selectivity for HDAC classes I and II [39, 40]. In a phase I study of 24 patients with advanced MDS (11 patients), AML (12 patients), and lymphoma (1 patient), pracinostat was generally well tolerated, demonstrated target inhibition, and showed preliminary clinical activity in 9 patients (1 CR, 1 PR /partial remission/, and 1 SD /stable disease/) [29]. A pilot phase 2 study was conducted as an extension of phase 1 study to determine the efficacy and safety of the combination of pracinostat with AZA in patients with MDS [29]. The ORR (CR, CR with incomplete blood count recovery /CRi/, and PR together) for the nine patients included in the study was 89%, and the CR with CRi rate was 78%. Grade 3/4 toxicities were neutropenic fever (22%) and thrombocytopenia (22%).

Panobinostat (LBH589) is a very potent panhistone HDACI currently being investigated in a number of human malignancies [41]. Two phase 2 non-randomized single arm trials of oral HDACI panobinostat were conducted in patients with low or intermediate-1 risk MDS [42, 43]. The objective of this study was to determine the clinical efficacy, safety, and tolerability of panobinostat in this patient population. The study would stop early if there was a chance >99% that the average overall response rate was <15%. Thirteen patients were treated. Median age was 70 years (range 47–84), 70% were transfusion dependent, 70% had intermediate-1 risk MDS. Most patients were diploid but one patient with del(5q), one with trisomy 8, one with complex cytogenetics, and two with deletion of 20q were included. Approximately 40% had previous therapy for MDS. Of the 13 patients, 1 (8%) achieved hematological improvement (duration 3 months) and 6 (46%) had stable disease for a median duration of 6 months (range 1.7–13.6). Treatment was withheld in one patient because of QTc prolongation but no other serious adverse effects were otherwise observed. In cardiology, the QT interval is a measure of the time between the start of the Q wave and the end of the T wave in the heart's electrical cycle. Modern computer-based ECG machines can easily calculate corrected QT (QTc). Panobinostat did not consistently induce histone acetylation as measured with Western blot. This data indicates that panobinostat at the dose and schedule studied has limited activity in lower risk MDS [42, 43].

A phase 1b/2 study was undertaken to evaluate the maximum-tolerated dose (MTD) and preliminary efficacy of the pan-HDACI panobinostat in combination with AZA in patients with AML or high-risk MDS naive to intensive chemotherapy [44]. Thirty-nine patients (AML=29, MDS=10) received AZA 75 mg/m^2) subcutaneously (days 1-5) and oral panobinostat (starting on day 5, thrice weekly for seven doses) in 28-day cycles until toxicity or disease progression. Dose-limiting toxicities during the phase 1b stage were observed in 0/4 patients receiving 10 mg panobinostat, in 1/7 patients (fatigue) receiving 20 mg, in 1/6 patients (fatigue) receiving 30 mg and in 4/5 patients (fatigue, syncope, hyponatremia and somnolence) receiving 40 mg. In phase 2, an additional 17 patients received panobinostat at a MTD of 30 mg. The most frequent AEs were fatigue (52%), injection site reaction (52%), nausea (30%), anorexia (30%), diarrhea (26%), and constipation (26%). Common grade 3/4 AEs included febrile neutropenia (22%), nausea (17%), dyspnea (17%), and infection (15%). The overall response rate (ORR=CR+CRi+PR) in patients with AML was 31% (9/29) and that in patients with MDS was 50% (5/10). After a median follow-up of 13 months, the median overall survival was 8 and 16 months in patients with AML and MDS, respectively. Increased histone H3 and H4 acetylation was a useful early biomarker of clinical response. Combining panobinostat with azacitidine was tolerable and clinically active in high-risk MDS/AML patients, warranting further exploration [44].

Open label phase II randomized trial comparing AZA 50 mg/m^2)/d given for 10 days ± entinostat 4 mg/m^2)/d day 3 and day 10 has been recently done [45]. All subtypes of myelodysplasia, chronic myelomonocytic leukemia, and AML with myelodysplasia-related changes were eligible for the study. The primary objective was the rate of hematologic normalization (HN; complete remission + partial remission + trilineage hematological improvement). One hundred forty-nine patients were analyzed, including 97 patients with MDS and 52 patients with AML. In the AZA group, 32% (95% CI /coincidence interval/, 22% to 44%) experienced HN and 27% (95% CI, 17% to 39%) in the AZA + entinostat group. Both arms exceeded the HN rate of historical control (Cancer and Leukemia Group B 9221 trial), but only the AZA group fulfilled the primary objective of the study. Rates of overall hematologic response were 46% and 44%, respectively. Median overall survivals were 18 months for the AZA group and 13 months for the AZA + entinostat group. The combination arm led to less demethylation compared with the monotherapy arm, suggesting pharmacodynamic antagonism. Addition of entinostat to AZA did not increase clinical response as defined by the protocol and was associated with pharmacodynamic antagonism [45]. However, the prolonged administration of AZA by itself seems to increase HN rate compared with standard dosing and warrants additional investigation.

Sequential administration of DNMT inhibitors and HDAC inhibitors has demonstrated clinical efficacy in patients with hematologic malignancies. However, the mechanism behind their clinical efficacy remains controversial. The methylation dynamics of 4 tumor suppressor genes /TSGs/ (p15^{INK4B} /cyclin-dependent kinase 4 inhibitor B/, CDH-1 /cadherin-1/, DAPK-1 /death-associated protein kinase 1/, and SOCS-1/suppressor of cytokine signaling 1/) were studied in sequential bone marrow samples from 30 patients with MDS or AML who completed a minimum of 4 cycles of therapy with 5-azacytidine and entinostat [46]. Reversal of promoter methylation after therapy was observed in both clinical responders and nonresponders across all genes. There was no association between clinical response and either baseline methylation or methylation reversal in the bone marrow or purified CD34$^+$ population, nor was there an association with change in gene expression. Transient global hypomethylation was observed in samples after treatment but was not associated with clinical response. Induction of histone H3/H4 acetylation and the DNA damage-associated variant histone γ-H2AX was observed in peripheral blood samples across all dose cohorts. In conclusion, methylation reversal of candidate TSGs during cycle 1 of therapy was not predictive of clinical response to combination "epigenetic" therapy [46].

HDACIS IN ACUTE MYELOID LEUKEMIA THERAPY

Two nonexclusive models have emerged to explain the establishment of pathological epigenetic changes [47]. In a stochastic model, overexpression of a given component of the machinery responsible for writing epigenetic code may cause deregulated expression of a gene important for tumorigenesis. This is consistent with experimental findings showing overexpression of some histone- and DNA- modifying enzymes in AML. HDACIs are a new class of drugs with significant antileukemic activity. To explore mechanisms of disease-specific HDACI activity in AML, the expression of all 18 members of the HDAC family in primary AML blasts and in four control cell types, namely $CD34^+$ progenitors from umbilical cord, either quiescent or cycling (post-culture), cycling $CD34^+$ progenitors from GCSF-stimulated adult donors and peripheral blood mononuclear cells was characterised [48]. Only SIRT1 was consistently overexpressed (>2 fold) in AML samples compared with all controls, while HDAC6 was overexpressed relative to adult, but not neo-natal cells. HDAC5 and SIRT4 were consistently underexpressed. AML blasts and cell lines, exposed to HDACIs in culture, showed both histone hyperacetylation and, unexpectedly, specific hypermethylation of H3 lysine 4. Such treatment also modulated the pattern of HDAC expression, with strong induction of HDAC11 in all myeloid cells tested and with all inhibitors (valproate, butyrate, TSA, SAHA), and lesser, more selective, induction of HDAC9 and SIRT4. The distinct pattern of HDAC expression in AML and its response to HDACIs is of relevance to the development of HDACI-based therapeutic strategies and may contribute to observed patterns of clinical response and development of drug resistance [48].

In the recruitment model, chromatin-modifying complexes are inappropriately targeted to regulatory regions of specific genes by fusion oncoproteins. This was shown to play a role in some subtypes of AML, such as AML1/ETO (also named RUNX1/RUNX1T1) and PML-retinoic acid receptor (RAR)α. The translocation (8;21)(q22;q22) is observed in approximately 12–15% of patients with AML, making it one of the most frequently observed translocations in AML [49]. Acute promyelocytic leukemia (APL) is characterized by an arrest of granulocytic differentiation and a reciprocal t(15;17) translocation fusing the PML gene to the retinoic acid receptor alpha (RARα) gene [50]. The fusion gene *CBFβ–MYH11* is created by the inv(16)(p13.1;q22) inversion and is associated with favorable prognosis in AML [51]. This chimeric gene *CBFβ–MYH11* encodes a fusion protein between CBFβ and smooth muscle myosin heavy chain (SMMHC/MYH11). This fusion protein causes the abberant recruitment of HDACs to promoters, resulting in a block in differentiation and uncontrolled proliferation of malignant cells [52, 53]. CBFB-MYH11 inhibits the RUNX1 activity. Whereas the AML1-ETO translocation is usually observed in AML subtype M2, the inversion of chromosome 16, inv(16)(p13q22), is associated with AML-M4Eo. In contrast to AML1, which recruits the transcriptional co-activators p300/CBP endowed with intrinsic HAT activity, AML1/ETO recruits, via NCoR/Sin3A, HDAC1 and the DNA methyltransferase-1 (DNMT1), resulting in the stable silencing of AML1-controlled genes, like those driving granulocytic maturation. The use of HDACIs to restore deregulated histone acetylation emerged as possible novel approach to AML therapy. Therefore, HDACIs are very potent anti-leukemic agents, particularly in AML1/ETO-positive cells [54]. The example of abberant recruitment of HDAC to fusion protein is shown in Figure 1 on example of the function of fusion proteins RUNX1-Evi1 and RUNX–MDS1-Evi1 in comparison with RUNX1.

Valproic acid and other HDACIs use in therapy of MDS and AML was described in previous paragraph about therapy in MDS. The same HDACIs were also tried in other studies connected with therapy of AML patients. Fredly et al. described the effects of VPA on AML cells and the clinical studies for combining VPA with other antileukemic agents [55, 56].

Vorinostat is a HDACI that has been shown to promote cell cycle arrest, growth inhibition, apoptosis and differentiation of cells from AML and MDS patients [57]. Vorinostat increased expression of genes down-regulated in MDS and/or AML (cFOS, COX2, IER3, p15, RAI3) and suppressed expression of genes over-expressed in these malignancies (AXL, c-MYC, Cyclin D1) and modulated cell cycle and apoptosis genes in a manner which would favor cell cycle arrest, differentiation, and apoptosis of neoplastic cells, consistent with the functional assays. Reporter assays showed transcriptional effect of vorinostat on some of these genes was mediated by proximal promoter elements in GC-rich regions. Vorinostat-modulated expression of some genes was potentiated by mithramycin A, a compound that interferes with transcription factor SP1 binding to GC-rich DNA sequences, and siRNA-mediated SP1 reduction. ChIP assays revealed vorinostat inhibited DNA binding of SP1 to the proximal promoter regions of these genes. These results suggest vorinostat transcriptional action in some genes is regulated by proximal promoter GC-rich DNA sequences and by SP1.

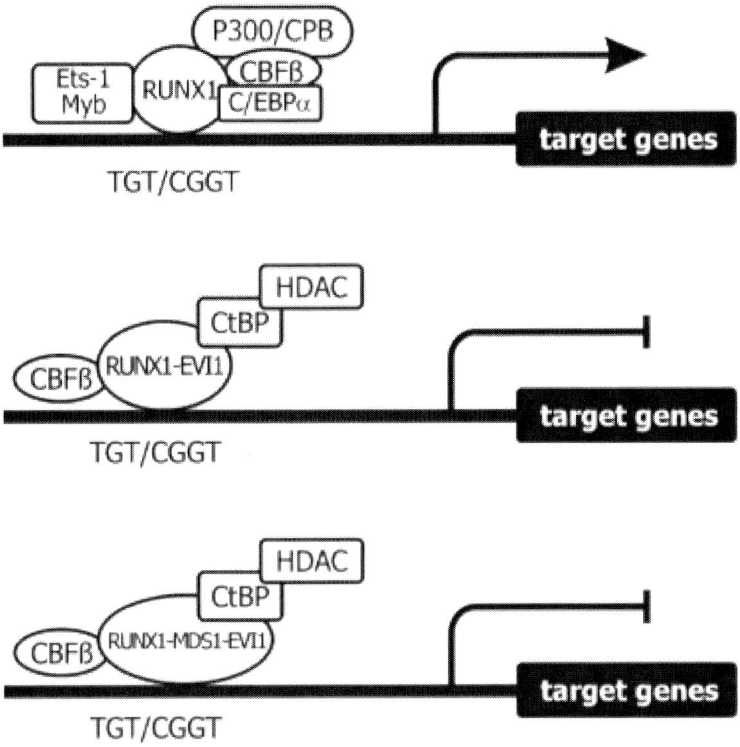

Figure 1. RUNX1 - CBFβ complex acts as RUNX1 target genes transcription activator, following interactions with other specific transcription factors, e.g., with Ets-1/Myb, C/EBPα and with transcription coactivator histone acetyltransferase (HAT), which are two nuclear phosphoproteins P300/CBP (CREB /cAMP response element/- binding protein). Contrary to that, RUNX1-EVI1 a RUNX1-MDS1-EVI1 fusion proteins act as RUNX1 target genes transcription supressors, as they bind to the CtBP transcription cosupressor and histone deacetylase.

An initial phase 2 study in 37 patients with relapsed or untreated AML, who were not candidates for chemotherapy, showed minimal activity in monotherapy [58]. A total dose of 8400 mg of vorinostat was delivered in each 21-day cycle of treatment: in arm A the dose regimen was 400 mg daily whereas in arm B the dose regimen was 200 mg three times daily for 14 days followed by 1 week rest. Data from all 37 patients were used for the analyses. In arm A (n=15), the confirmed complete remission rate was 0% (95% CI, 0%

to 23%); this arm was closed at the planned interim analysis. In arm B (n=22), the confirmed complete remission rate was 4.5% (1 response; 95% CI, 0.4% to 24%), with a duration of response exceeding 398 days. The median time to treatment failure in arm A was 42 days (95% CI, 26 to 57); although a minimum of four cycles of treatment were planned, 11 patients (79%) received no more than two cycles. The median time to treatment failure in arm B was 46 days (95% CI, 20 to 71); 13 patients (59%) received no more than two cycles of treatment. Therapy was discontinued in many patients before the planned four cycles had been administered, either because of failure of vorinostat to control the leukocyte count or patients' and physicians' preference. Future studies of vorinostat in AML should focus on combinations with other drugs with which it might interact pharmacodynamically.

This led to several combination trials. A phase 2 study of vorinostat in combination with gemtuzumab ozogamicin (GO) has been completed in the setting of older adults with untreated AML [59]. Patients were stratified into 2 groups (group 1: patients aged ≥ 70 years and performance status 2-3; group 2: aged 60-69 years with performance status 0-3 or aged ≥ 70 years and performance status 0-1). Responses were monitored separately in group 2 patients with normal or favorable cytogenetics (group 2A) and other cytogenetics (group 2B). Among 31 patients, 6 (19.4%) achieved complete remission, and one (3.2%) achieved complete remission with incomplete platelet recovery; these patients had a higher median overall survival than non-responders (553 vs. 131 days, P = 0.0026). Response rates were: group 1, one of 10 (10.0%); group 2A, 6 of 13 (46.2%); and group 2B, none of 8 (0%). These data indicate that vorinostat+GO has activity that is mostly confined to patients with normal karyotype disease.

Epigenetic therapeutics such as the histone deacetylase inhibitor, vorinostat, and the DNA methyltransferase I inhibitor, azacitidine, enhance GO efficacy in vitro. Therefore, a combination vorinostat/azacitidine/ gemtuzumab ozogamicin has been investigated in 52 adults aged 50 years or over with AML requiring therapy for first relapse (remission duration ≤ 12 months) or primary refractory disease in a phase 1/2 trial [60]. Vorinostat and GO were escalated step-wise during the phase I portion of the trial. Vorinostat (400 mg/day orally from Days 1-9), azacitidine (75 mg/m(2)/day intravenously or subcutaneously from Days 1-7), and GO (3 mg/m(2)/day intravenously on Days 4 and 8) were identified as the maximum tolerated dose. Among the 43 patients treated at this dose, 10 achieved a complete remission and 8 achieved a complete remission with incomplete blood count recovery, for an overall response rate of 41.9% (exact 95% confidence interval (CI): 27.0-57.9%).

Four of these 18 patients (2 with complete remission and 2 with complete remission with incomplete blood count recovery) had persistence of minimal residual disease by flow cytometry at the time of best response. Four patients died within 28 days of treatment initiation. Median overall survival for the 18 patients achieving complete remission/complete remission with incomplete blood count recovery was significantly longer than for those 21 patients who failed therapy but lived at least 29 days after treatment initiation (224.5 days (range 70-798) vs. 95 days (range 36-900); P=0.0023). These data indicate that vorinostat/azacitidine/gemtuzumab ozogamicin has activity in this difficult-to-treat AML patient subset [60].

Another HDACI panobinostat seems to potentiate the antileukemic effect of fludarabine [61] and sensitizes leukemic blasts to cytarabine and daunorubicin [62]. Oral panobinostat is also studied in combination with azacitidine in adult patients with AML or MDS [44, 63]. AML provides an environment that enables immune suppression, resulting in functionally defective effector T cells. Regulatory T cells (Treg) are significant contributors to the impaired antitumor immune response. As tumor necrosis factor (TNF) is present at high levels in AML and TNF receptor-2 (TNFR2)-expressing Tregs identify highly functional Tregs, the hypothesis that $TNFR2^+$ Tregs are a relevant Treg subset in this cancer was investigated. We also determine the effect of the novel combinatorial therapy of the demethylating agent, azacitidine with the HDACI, panobinostat on Tregs, particularly $TNFR2^+$ Tregs [63]. $TNFR2^+$ Tregs are increased in AML and have a high migration potential toward the bone marrow. Furthermore, the level of $TNFR2^+$ Tregs in the peripheral blood and the bone marrow of patients was shown decreased in vivo after exposure to panobinostat and azacitidine. Reductions in $TNFR2^+$ Tregs were associated with increases in interferon (IFN)-γ and interleukin (IL)-2 production by effector T cells within the bone marrow and beneficial clinical responses. In vitro mechanistic studies indicated panobinostat as the primary driver for the reduction of Tregs. Our study provides for the first time, in vivo validation of the ability of panobinostat in combination with azacitidine to suppress prevalent $TNFR2^+$ Tregs, resulting in clinical benefits within patients with AML.

Pracinostat (SB939), an oral HDACI with single-agent activity in MDS and AML [40, 64, 65], showed promising results in a phase 2 study in combination with azacitidine [66].

HDACIS IN CHRONIC MYELOID LEUKEMIA THERAPY

In chronic myelocytic leukemia (CML) the activity of the Bcr-Abl tyrosine kinase is known to activate a number of molecular mechanisms, which inhibit apoptosis. The histone deacetylase inhibitor SAHA (suberoylanilide hydroxamic acid, vorinostat) markedly decreases protein expression levels of Bcr-Abl and c-Myc in BV-173 cells, while in K562 cells only a minor decrease of Bcr-Abl protein levels is observed while a considerable reduction of c-Myc protein expression may only be achieved at higher concentrations of SAHA [67]. BV-173 cells were more sensitive to SAHA-induced apoptosis when compared to K562 cells. Even though earlier reports on SAHA considerably focused on its inhibitory effect on HDAC enzymatic activity, we report herein a significant down-regulation of HDAC3 protein expression levels following treatment with SAHA in BV-173 cells, but not in K562 cells. In conclusion, our results imply a molecular mechanism for SAHA-induced apoptosis in BV-173 cells, which involves decreased protein expression levels of Bcr-Abl, c-Myc and HDAC3.

Treatment with LAQ824 (Novartis Pharmaceutical, Inc.), a cinnamyl hydroxamic acid analogue inhibitor of histone deacetylases, depleted the mRNA and protein expression of Bcr-Abl in human chronic myeloid leukemia blast crisis (CML-BC) cells [68]. Exposure to LAQ824 induced the expression of the cell cycle-dependent kinase inhibitors p21 and p27 and caused cell cycle G(1)-phase accumulation and apoptosis of CML-BC cells. LAQ824 also induced acetylation of heat shock protein 90. This inhibited the chaperone association of Bcr-Abl with heat shock protein 90, thereby promoting the proteasomal degradation of Bcr-Abl. Cotreatment with LAQ824 increased imatinib mesylate-induced apoptosis of CML-BC cells. Additionally, LAQ824 down-regulated the levels of mutant Bcr-Abl possessing the T315I point mutation, as well as induced apoptosis of imatinib-refractory primary CML-BC cells. Therefore, LAQ824 may be a promising therapeutic agent in the treatment of imatinib-sensitive or -refractory human leukemia [68].

Resistance to imatinib (Gleevec®) in cancer cells is frequently because of acquired point mutations in the kinase domain of BCR-ABL. Ponatinib, also known as AP24534, is an oral multi-targeted tyrosine kinase inhibitor (TKI), and it has been investigated in a pivotal phase 2 clinical trial. The histone deacetylase inhibitor vorinostat (suberoylanilide hydroxamic acid) has been evaluated for its significant clinical activity in hematological malignancies. Thus, treatments combining ABL TKIs with additional drugs may be a promising strategy in the treatment of leukemia. The efficacy of ponatinib and vorinostat treatment was analyzed by using BCR-ABL-positive cell lines [69]. Treatment with ponatinib for 72 h inhibited cell growth and induced apoptosis in K562 cells in a dose-dependent manner. Ponatinib potently inhibited the growth of Ba/F3 cells ectopically expressing BCR-ABL T315I mutation. Upon BCR-ABL phosphorylation, Crk-L was decreased, and poly (ADP-ribose) polymerase (PARP) was activated in a dose-dependent manner. CRKL is a major substrate of the deregulated BCR/ABL tyrosine kinase and is aberrantly tyrosine-phosphorylated in Ph-positive leukemia cells. Combined treatment of Ba/F3 T315I mutant cells with vorinostat and ponatinib resulted in significantly increased cytotoxicity. Additionally, the intracellular signaling of ponatinib and vorinostat was examined. Caspase 3 and PARP activation increased after combination treatment with ponatinib and vorinostat. Moreover, an increase in the phosphorylation levels of γH2A.X was observed. Previously established ponatinib-resistant Ba/F3 cells were also resistant to imatinib, nilotinib, and dasatinib. We investigated the difference in the efficacy of ponatinib and vorinostat by using ponatinib-resistant Ba/F3 cells. Combined treatment of ponatinib-resistant cells with ponatinib and vorinostat caused a significant increase in cytotoxicity. Thus, combined administration of ponatinib and vorinostat may be a powerful strategy against BCR-ABL mutant cells and could enhance the cytotoxic effects of ponatinib in those BCR-ABL mutant cells [69].

The HDAC inhibitors vorinostat and/or pracinostat (SB939) induced apoptosis in BCR-ABL-expressing cells [70]. Additionally, HDAC inhibitors reduced levels of Aurora A and B protein. An Aurora kinase inhibitor, tozasertib (VX-680), inhibited growth, promoted pro-apoptotic activity, reduced the phosphorylation of BCR-ABL and Crk-L, and activated caspase-3 and poly (ADP-ribose) polymerase (PARP) in BCR-ABL-positive cells. Moreover, after treatment with tozasertib, HDAC protein expression was decreased. Combination of vorinostat or pracinostat with tozasertib had a synergistic inhibitory effect on the proliferation of T315I cells. Phosphorylation of Crk-L decreased, and PARP activation increased after treatment with vorinostat or pracinostat and tozasertib. Moreover, combination of vorinostat or pracinostat and tozasertib significantly increased the extent of apoptosis in primary CML cells [70].

HDACIs in Other Chronic Myeloproliferative Neoplasm Therapy

Myeloproliferative neoplasms (MPN) are clonal haemopoietic progenitor cell disorders characterized by the proliferation of one or more of the haemopoietic lineages (myeloid, erythroid and/or megakaryocytic). The MPNs include eight haematological disorders: CML, polycythemia vera (PV), essential thrombocythemia (ET), primary myelofibrosis (PMF), systemic mastocytosis (SM), chronic eosinophilic leukemia, not otherwise specified (CEL, NOS), chronic neutrophilic leukemia (CNL), and unclassifiable MPN (MPN, U). The BCR-ABL1-negative MPNs include polycythemia vera, essential thrombocythemia, and primary myelofibrosis. Therapeutic interventions for MPNs include the use of tyrosine kinase inhibitors (TKIs) for BCR-ABL1$^+$ CML and JAK2 inhibitors for PV, ET and PMF. HDACIs are a novel class of drugs capable of altering the acetylation status of both histone and non-histone proteins, thereby affecting a repertoire of cellular functions in neoplastic cells including proliferation, differentiation, immune responses, angiogenesis and survival. Preliminary studies indicate that HDACIs when used in combination with tyrosine kinase or JAK2 inhibitors may overcome resistance to the latter agents and enhance the pro-apoptotic effects on MPN cells [71, 72].

Polycythemia vera (PV) is a chronic myeloproliferative neoplasm defined by erythrocytosis and often accompanied by leukocytosis and thrombocytosis. Current treatment options, including IFN-α and hydroxyurea, effectively manage PV in many patients. However, some high-risk patients, particularly those who become hydroxyurea-intolerant/resistant, may benefit from IFN-α or new treatment options. A better understanding of PV pathophysiology, including the role of the JAK/STAT pathway, has inspired the development of new therapies. Several JAK inhibitors directly target JAK/STAT pathway activation and have been evaluated in Phase II/III trials with promising results. Pegylated variants of IFN-α, which reduce dosing frequency and toxicity associated with recombinant IFN-α, have yielded favorable efficacy results in Phase II trials. Finally, histone deacetylase inhibitors have been developed to manage PV at the level of chromatin-regulated gene expression [73]. The earliest Phase III results from these next-generation therapies are expected in 2014.

Panobinostat, a pan-deacetylase inhibitor that depletes JAK2 V617F levels and JAK/STAT signalling in MPN cells, was evaluated in patients with primary MF, post-essential thrombocythaemia MF, and post-polycythaemia vera MF [74, 75]. Patients received panobinostat 20-40 mg administered three times per week [74, 75]. Dose reductions were permitted for toxicities. The primary endpoint was response rate at 6 months using International Working Group for Myelofibrosis Research and Treatment (IWG-MRT) consensus criteria. Analyses of peripheral blood cells from treated patients revealed that panobinostat inhibited JAK/STAT signalling, decreased inflammatory cytokine levels, and decreased JAK2 V617F allelic burden. However, panobinostat was poorly tolerated at the dose and schedule evaluated, and only 16 of 35 patients completed ≥2 cycles of treatment. One patient (3%) achieved an IWG-MRT response. Common adverse events were thrombocytopenia (71.4%) and diarrhoea (80.0%). Although molecular correlative analyses suggested that panobinostat inhibits key intracellular targets, limited clinical activity was observed because of poor tolerance.

Vorinostat 400 mg was administered once daily for 24 weeks after which patients were observed for an additional 12 weeks without vorinostat. Patients who required dose modification to less than 300 mg were withdrawn from the study. Hydroxyurea was permitted to control platelet count if the patient developed ischemic symptoms. Fourteen patients (11 primary myelofibrosis (PMF) and 3 post-polycythemia vera myelofibrosis (PPV-MF) were included in the study [76]. Eight patients (57%) were followed to hospital visit n. 8 (i.e., end of intervention period). Five of these patients had been treated with vorinostat as monotherapy and the other 3 had also received concomitant HU. An intention-to-treat (ITT) response rate of 14% was observed: 2 of 14 patients, one in complete remission (CR) and one with clinical improvement (CI). None of the concomitantly treated patients experienced a clinical response at the end of intervention.

Conclusion and Perspectives

HDACIs are a relative new class of anti-cancer agents that play important roles in epigenetic or non-epigenetic regulation. HDACIs induce death, apoptosis, and cell cycle arrest in cancer cells. Most of the published clinical trials of HDACIs in MDS and AML are phase 1. As single agents the response rates observed have been relatively low, usually between 10 and 20% [12]. Toxicities with these agents demonstrate a common patern and include fatigue, nausea, vomiting, and diarrhea. Although most of these studies evaluated the correlative endpoint of histone acetylation, no associations between hyperacetylation of histones and response to therapy have been demonstrated. Development of novel therapies is connected with the development of new combinations of these agents with other anti-cancer therapeutics, to improve response rates and durability of responses. There has been significant enthusiasm for a combination of azanucleotides (azacitidine and decitabine) with HDACIs. These combinations resulted in synergistic re-expression of DNA methylation silenced genes *in vitro* [22]. Combined DNA methyltransferase and histone deacetylase inhibition showed a higher response rate than for single agent also in clinical studies [37, 45]. Some studies with these combinations failed to substantiate a correlaton between gene specific reversal of methylation and response [23, 46]. The combination of HDACIs and proteasome inhibitors is useful in the treatment of human myeloid leukemia especially in the context of molecular targeted therapy [77-79]. Despite the considerable efficacy of these combinations, patients with underlying myelo-dysplasia continue to have a remarkably poor outcome and novel strategies in these diseases remain essential. The fusion oncoproteins PML-RARα and BCR-ABL, the main oncogenic drivers of APL and CML, respectively, have recently been identified as autophagy substrates and their degradation by autophagy shown to contribute to treatment. However, this does not seem to be a general feature of leukemic fusion oncoproteins, as AML1/ETO fusion protein is not an autophagy substrate. The constitutive suppression of autophagy due to mTOR activation represents an inherent difference between cancer and normal cells. Thus, via autophagy suppression, HDACIs deprive cells of an essential pro-survival mechanism [17]. Gene expression profiling and epigenome studies during treatment with HDACIs are ongoing in an attempt to clarify particular patterns of gene and epigenome deregulation that is necessary for a better understanding of clinical and biochemical effects of HDACIs.

ACKNOWLEDGEMENTS

This work was supported by research project (Ministry of Health, Czech Republic) for conceptual development of research organization (00023736; Institute of Hematology and Blood Transfusion, Prague).

REFERENCES

[1] Jenuwein, T; Allis, CD. Translating the histone code. ***Science***., 2001, 293, 1074-1080.

[2] Cosgrove, MS; Boeke, JD; Wolberger, C. Regulated nucleosome mobility and the histone code. *Nat. Struct. Mol. Biol*., 2004, 11, 1037-1043.

[3] Bannister, AJ; Kouzarides, T. Regulation of chromatin by histone modifications. *Cell Res.,* 2011, 21, 381-395.

[4] Rando, OJ. Combinatorial complexity in chromatin structure and function: revisiting the histone code. *Curr. Opin. Genet. Dev.,* 2012, 22, 148-155.

[5] Lakshmaiah, KC; Jacob, LA; Aparna, S; Lokanatha, D; Saldanha, SC. Epigenetic therapy of cancer with histone deacetylase inhibitors. *J. Cancer Res. Ther*. 2014, 10, 469-478.

[6] Kouraklis, G; Misiakos, EP; Theocharis, S. Histone deacetylase inhibitors as a potential therapeutic agent for human cancer treatment. *Targ. Oncol.,* 2006, 1, 34-41.

[7] Xu, WS; Parmigiani, RB; Marks, PA. Histone deacetylase inhibitors: molecular mechanisms of action. *Oncogene,* 2007, 26, 5541-5552.

[8] Gore, SD; Hermes-De Santis, ER. Future directions in myelodysplastic syndrome: newer agents and the role of combination approaches. *Cancer Control*, 2008, 15 (Suppl), 40-49.

[9] Frew, AJ; Johnstone, RW; Bolden, JE. Enhancing the apoptotic and therapeutic effects of HDAC inhibitors. *Cancer Lett.,* 2009, 280, 125-133.

[10] Tambaro, FP; Dell'Aversana, C; Carafa, V; Nebbioso, A; Radic, B; Ferrara, F; Altucci, L. Histone deacetylase inhibitors: clinical implications for hematological malignancies. *Clin Epigenet.,* 2010, 1, 25-44.

[11] Marks, PA. Histone deacetylase inhibitors: A chemical genetics approach to understanding cellular functions. *Biochim. Biophys. Acta,* 2010, 1799, 717-725.

[12] Quintás-Cardama, A; Santos, FP; Garcia-Manero, G. Histone deacetylase inhibitors for the treatment of myelodysplastic syndrome and acute myeloid leukemia. *Leukemia,* 2011, 25, 226-235.

[13] Prebet, T; Vey, N. Vorinostat in acute myeloid leukemia and myelodysplastic syndromes. *Expert Opin. Investig. Drugs,* 2011, 20, 287-295.

[14] Bose, P; Dai, Y; Grant, S. Histone deacetylase inhibitor (HDACI) mechanisms of action: emerging insights. *Pharmacol. Therapeut.,* 2014, 323-336, 2014.

[15] Li, Z; Zhu, WG. Targeting histone deacetylases for cancer therapy: from molecular mechanisms to clinical implications. *Int. J. Biol. Sci.,* 2014, 10, 757-770.

[16] Kroesen, M; Gielen, PR; Brok, IC; Armandari, I; Hoogerbrugge, PM; Adema, GJ. HDAC inhibitors and immunotherapy; a double edged sword? *Oncotarget,* 2014, 5, 6558-6572.

[17] Stankov, MV; El Khatib, M; Kumar Thakur, B; Heitmann, K; Panayotova-Dimitrova, D; Schoening, J; Bourquin, JP; Schweitzer, N; Leverkus, M; Welte, K; Reinhardt, D; Li, Z; Orkin, SH; Behrens, GM; Klusmann, JH. Histone deacetylase inhibitors induce apoptosis in myeloid leukemia by suppressing autophagy. *Leukemia,* 2014, 28, 577-588.

[18] Rasheed, WK; Johnstone, RW; Prince, HM. Histone deacetylase inhibitors in cancer therapy. *Expert Opin. Investig. Drugs,* 2007, 16, 659-678.

[19] Dokmanovic, M; Clarke, C; Marks, PA. Histone deacetylase inhibitors: overview and perspectives. *Mol. Cancer Res.*, 2007, 5, 981-989.

[20] Marks, PA; Breslow, R. Dimethyl sulfoxide to vorinostat: development of this histone deacetylase inhibitor as an anticancer drug. *Nat. Biotechnol.,* 2007, 25, 84-90.

[21] Glaser, KB. HDAC inhibitors: clinical update and mechanism-based potential. *Biochem. Pharmacol.*, 2007, 74, 659-671.

[22] Cameron, EE; Bachman, KE; Myöhänen, S; Herman, JG; Baylin, SB. Synergy of demethylation and histone deacetylase inhibition in the re-expression of genes silence in cancer. *Nat. Genet.*, 1999, 21, 103-107.

[23] Gore, SD; Baylin, S; Sugar, E; Carraway, H; Miller, CB; Carducci, M; Grever, M; Galm, O; Dauses, T; Karp, JE; Rudek, MA; Zhao, M; Smith, BD; Manning, J; Jiemjit, A; Dover, G; Mays, A; Zwiebel, J; Murgo, A; Weng, LJ; Herman, JG. Combined, DNA methyltransferase and histone deacetylase inhibition in the treatment of myeloid neoplasm. *Cancer Res.,* 2006, 66, 6361-6369.

[24] Garcia-Manero, G; Kantarjian, HM; Sanchez-Gonzales, B; Yang, H; Rosner, G; Verstovsek, S; Rytting, M; Wierda, WG; Ravandi, F; Koller, C; Xiao, L; Faderl, S; Estrov, Z; Cortes, J; O'brien, S; Estey, E; Bueso-Ramos, C; Fiorentino, J; Jabbour, E; Issa, JP. Phase 1/2 study of the

combination of 5-aza-2'-deoxycytidine with valproic acid in patients with leukemia. *Blood,* 2006, 108, 3271-3279.

[25] Soriano, AO; Yang, H; Faderl, S; Estrov, Z; Giles, F; Ravandi, F; Cortes, J; Wierda, WG; Ouzounian, S; Quezada, A; Pierce, S; Estey, EH; Issa, JP; Kantarjian, HM; Garcia-Manero, G. Safety and clinical activity of the combination of 5-azacytidine, valproic acid, and all-trans retinoic acid in acute myeloid leukemia and myelodysplastic syndrome. *Blood,* 2007, 110, 2302-2308.

[26] Lübbert, M. Epigenetic therapy for myelodysplastic syndromes has entered center stage. *Leuk. Res.*, 2009, 33, S27-S28.

[27] Abujamra, AL; Pinheiro dos Santos, M; Roesler, R; Schwartsmann, G; Brunnetto, AL. Histone deacetylase inhibitors: A new perspective for the treatment of leukemia. *Leuk. Res.,* 2010, 34, 687-695.

[28] Anargyrou, K; Vassilakopoulos, TP; Angelopoulou, M.K; Terpos, E. Incorporating novel agents in the treatment of myelodysplastic syndromes. *Leuk. Res.,* 2010, 34, 6-17.

[29] Jabbour, E; Garcia-Manero, G. Deacetylase Inhibitors for the Treatment of Myelodysplastic Syndromes. *Leuk. Lymphoma*, 2014, Jul 24,1-26; DOI: 10.3109/10428194.2014.946025.

[30] Garcia-Manero, G; Yang, H; Bueso-Ramos, C; Ferrajoli, A; Cortes, J; Wierda, WG; Faderl, S; Koller, C; Morris, G; Rosner, G; Loboda, A; Fantin, VR; Randolph, SS; Hardwick, JS; Reilly, JF; Chen, C; Ricker, JL; Secrist, JP; Richon, VM; Frankel, SR; Kantarjian, HM. Phase 1 study of the histone deacetylase inhibitor vorinostat (suberoylanilide hydroxamic acid [SAHA]) in patients with advanced leukemias and myelodysplastic syndromes. *Blood,* 2008,111, 1060-1066.

[31] Garcia-Manero, G; Tambaro, FP; Bekele, NB; Yang, H; Ravandi, F; Jabbour, E; Borthakur, G; Kadia, TM; Konopleva, MY; Faderl, S; Cortes, JE; Brandt, M; Hu, Y; McCue, D; Newsome, WM; Pierce, SR; de Lima, M; Kantarjian, HM. Phase II trial of vorinostat with idarubicin and cytarabine for patients with newly diagnosed acute myelogenous leukemia or myelodysplastic syndrome. *J. Clin. Oncol.*, 2012, 30, 2204-2210.

[32] Klimek, VM; Fircanis, S; Maslak, P; Guernah, I; Baum, M; Wu, N; Panageas, K; Wright, JJ; Pandolfi, PP; Nimer, SD. Tolerability, pharmacodynamics, and pharmacokinetics studies of depsipeptide (romidepsin) in patients with acute myelogenous leukemia or advanced myelodysplastic syndromes. *Clin. Cancer Res.*, 2008, 14, 826-832.

[33] Kuendgen, A; Gattermann, N. Valproic acid for the treatment of myeloid malignancies. *Cancer,* 2007, 110, 943-954.

[34] Kuendgen, A; Strupp, C; Aivado, M; Bernhardt, A; Hildebrandt, B; Haas, R; Germing, U; Gattermann, N. Treatment of myelodysplastic syndromes with valproic acid alone or in combination with all-trans retinoic acid. *Blood,* 2004, 104, 1266-1269.

[35] Cortes, J. Treatment of myelodysplastic syndromes with valproic acid alone or in combination with all-trans retinoic acid. *Curr. Hematol. Rep.*, 2005, 4, 173-174.

[36] Kuendgen, A; Knipp, S; Fox, F; Strupp, C; Hildebrandt, B; Steidl, C; Germing, U; Haas, R; Gattermann, N. Results of a phase 2 study of valproic acid alone or in combination with all-trans retinoic acid in 75 patients with myelodysplastic syndrome and relapsed or refractory acute myeloid leukemia. *Ann. Hematol.*, 2005, 84 (Suppl 1), 61-66.

[37] Blum, W; Klisovic, RB; Hackanson, B; Liu, Z; Liu, S; Devine, H; Vukosavljevic, T; Huynh, L; Lozanski, G; Kefauver, C; Plass, C; Devine, SM; Heerema, NA; Murgo, A; Chan, KK; Grever, MR; Byrd, JC; Marcucci, G. Phase I study of decitabine alone or in combination with valproic acid in acute myeloid leukemia. *J. Clin. Oncol.*, 2007, 25, 3884-3891.

[38] Kuendgen, A; Bug, G; Ottmann, OG; Haase, D; Schanz, J; Hildebrandt, B; Nachtkamp, K; Neukirchen, J; Dienst, A; Haas, R; Germing, U; Gattermann, N. Treatment of poor-risk myelodysplastic syndromes and acute myeloid leukemia with a combination of 5-azacytidine and valproic acid. *Clin. Epigenetics,* 2011, 2, 389-399.

[39] Novotny-Diermayr, V; Sangthongpitag, K; Hu, CY; Wu, X; Sausgruber, N; Yeo, P; Greicius, G; Pettersson, S; Liang, AL; Loh, YK; Bonday, Z; Goh, KC; Hentze, H; Hart, S; Wang, H; Ethirajulu, K; Wood, JM. SB939, a novel potent and orally active histone deacetylase inhibitor with high tumor exposure and efficacy in mouse models of colorectal cancer. *Mol. Cancer Ther.,* 2010, 9, 642-652.

[40] Novotny-Diermayr, V; Hart, S; Goh, KC; Cheong, A; Ong, LC; Hentze, H; Pasha, MK; Jayaraman, R; Ethirajulu, K; Wood, JM. The oral HDAC inhibitor pracinostat (SB939) is efficacious and synergistic with the JAK2 inhibitor pacritinib (SB1518) in preclinical models of AML. *Blood Cancer J.,* 2011, 1, e44.

[41] Giles, F; Fischer, T; Cortes, J; et al. A phase I study of intravenous LBH589, a novel cinnamic hydroxamic acid analogue histone

deacetylase inhibitor, in patients with refractory hematologic malignancies. *Clin. Cancer Res*., 2006, 12, 4628–4635.

[42] Dimicoli, S; Jabbour, E; Borthakur, G; Kadia, T; Estrov, Z; Yang, H; Kelly, M; Pierce, S; Kantarjian, H; Garcia-Manero, G. Phase II study of the histone deacetylase inhibitor panobinostat (LBH589) in patients with low or intermediate-1 risk myelodysplastic syndrome. *Am. J. Hematol*., 2012, 87, 127-129.

[43] Platzbecker, U; Al-Ali, HK, Gattermann, N; Haase, D; Janzen, V; Krauter, J; Götze, K; Schlenk, R; Nolte, F; Letsch, A; Ottmann, OG; Kündgen, A; Lübbert, M; Germing, U; Wermke, M; Reinhard, H; Weiss, C; Lieder, K; Ehninger, G; Leismann, O; Giagounidis, A. Phase 2 study of oral panobinostat (LBH589) with or without erythropoietin in heavily transfusion-dependent IPSS low or int-1 MDS patients. *Leukemia* 2014, 28, 696-698.

[44] Tan, P; Wei, A; Mithraprabhu, S; Cummings, N; Liu, HB; Perugini, M; Reed, K; Avery, S; Patil, S; Walker, P; Mollee, P; Grigg, A; D'Andrea, R; Dear, A; Spencer, A. Dual epigenetic targeting with panobinostat and azacitidine in acute myeloid leukemia and high-risk myelodysplastic syndrome. *Blood Cancer J*., 2014, 10, e170.

[45] Prebet, T; Sun, Z; Figueroa, ME; Ketterling, R; Melnick, A; Greenberg, PL; Herman, J; Juckett, M; Smith, MR; Malick, L; Paietta, E; Czader, M; Litzow, M; Gabrilove, J; Erba, HP; Gore, SD; Tallman, MS. Prolonged administration of azacitidine with or without entinostat for myelodysplastic syndrome and acute myeloid leukemia with myelodysplasia-related changes: results of the US Leukemia Intergroup trial E1905. *J. Clin. Oncol*., 2014, 32, 1242-1248.

[46] Fandy, TE; Herman, JG; Kerns, P; Jiemjit, A; Sugar, EA; Choi, SH; Yang, AS; Aucott, T; Dauses, T; Odchimar-Reissig, R; Licht, J; McConnell, MJ; Nasrallah, C; Kim, MK; Zhang, W; Sun, Y; Murgo, A; Espinoza-Delgado, I; Oteiza, K; Owoeye, I; Silverman, LR; Gore, SD; Carraway, HE. Early epigenetic changes and DNA damage do not predict clinical response in an overlapping schedule of 5-azacytidine and entinostat in patients with myeloid malignancies. *Blood,* 2009, 114, 2764-2773.

[47] Zelent, A; Petrie, K; Lotan, R; Waxman, S; Gore, SD. Clinical translation of epigenetics in cancer: eN-CORe - a report on the second workshop. *Mol. Cancer Ther*., 2005, 4, 1810-1819.

[48] Bradbury, CA; Khanim, FL; Hayden, R; Bunce, CM; White, DA; Drayson, MT; Craddock, C; Turner, BM. Histone deacetylases in acute

myeloid leukaemia show a distinctive pattern of expression that changes selectively in response to deacetylase inhibitors. *Leukemia,* 2005, 19, 1751-1759.

[49] Peterson, LF; Zhang, DE. The 8; 21 translocation in leukemogenesis. *Oncogene,* 2004, 23, 4255–4262.

[50] Rousselot, P; Hardas, B; Patel, A; Guidez, F; Gäken, J; Castaigne, S; Dejean, A; de Thé, H; Degos, L; Farzaneh, F; et al. The PML-RAR alpha gene product of the t(15;17) translocation inhibits retinoic acid-induced granulocytic differentiation and mediated transactivation in human myeloid cells. *Oncogene,* 1994, 9, 545-551.

[51] Tobal, K; Johnson, PR; Saunders, MJ; Harrison, CJ; Liu Yin, JA. Detection of CBFB/MYH11 transcripts in patients with inversion and other abnormalities of chromosome 16 at presentation and remission. *Br. J. Haematol.*, 1995, 91, 104-108.

[52] Peloquin, GL; Chen, YB; Fathi, AT. The evolving landscape in the therapy of acute myeloid leukemia. *Protein Cell,* 2013, 4, 735-746.

[53] Mandoli, A; Singh, AA; Jansen, PW; Wierenga, AT; Riahi, H; Franci, G; Prange, K; Saeed, S; Vellenga, E; Vermeulen, M; Stunnenberg, HG; Martens, JH. CBFB-MYH11/RUNX1 together with a compendium of hematopoietic regulators, chromatin modifiers and basal transcription factors occupies self-renewal genes in inv(16) acute myeloid leukemia. *Leukemia,* 2014, 28, 770-778.

[54] Barbetti, V; Gozzini, A; Cheloni, G; Marzi, I; Fabiani, E; Santini, V; Dello Sbarba, P; Rovida, E. Time- and residue-specific differences in histone acetylation induced by VPA and SAHA in AML1/ETO-positive leukemia cells. *Epigenetics,* 2013, 8, 210-219.

[55] Fredly, H; Gjertsen, BT; Bruserud, O. Histone deacetylase inhibition in the treatment of acute myeloid leukemia: the effects of valproic acid on leukemic cells, and the clinical and experimental evidence for combining valproic acid with other antileukemic agents. *Clin. Epigenetics,* 2013, 5, 12.

[56] Fredly, H; Ersvær, E; Kittang, AO; Tsykunova, G; Gjertsen, BT; Bruserud, O. The combination of valproic acid, all-trans retinoic acid and low-dose cytarabine as disease-stabilizing treatment in acute myeloid leukemia. *Clin. Epigenetics,* 2013, 5, 13.

[57] Silva, G; Cardoso, BA; Belo, H; Almeida, AM. Vorinostat induces apoptosis and differentiation in myeloid malignancies: genetic and molecular mechanisms. *PLoS One,* 2013, 8, e53766.

[58] Schaefer, EW; Loaiza-Bonilla, A; Juckett, M; DiPersio, JF; Roy, V; Slack, J; Wu, W; Laumann, K; Espinoza-Delgado, I; Gore, SD; Mayo, P2C Phase II Consortium. A phase 2 study of vorinostat in acute myeloid leukemia. *Haematologica,* 2009, 94, 1375-1382.

[59] Walter, RB; Medeiros, BC; Powell, BL; Schiffer, CA; Appelbaum, FR; Estey, EH. Phase II trial of vorinostat and gemtuzumab ozogamicin as induction and post-remission therapy in older adults with previously untreated acute myeloid leukemia. *Haematologica,* 2012, 97, 739-742.

[60] Walter, RB; Medeiros, BC; Gardner, KM; Orlowski, KF; Gallegos, L; Scott, BL; Hendrie, PC; Estey, EH. Gemtuzumab ozogamicin in combination with vorinostat and azacitidine in older patients with relapsed or refractory acute myeloid leukemia: a phase I/II study. *Haematologica,* 2014, 99, 54-59.

[61] Rosato, R; Hock, S; Dent, P; Dai, Y; Grant, S. LBH-589 (panobinostat) potentiates fludarabine anti-leukemic activity through a JNK- and XIAP-dependent mechanism. *Leuk. Res.,* 2012, 36, 491-498.

[62] Xie, C; Drenberg, C; Edwards, H; Caldwell, JT; Chen, W; Inaba, H; Xu, X; Buck, SA; Taub, JW; Baker, SD; Ge, Y. Panobinostat enhances cytarabine and daunorubicin sensitivities in AML cells through suppressing the expression of BRCA1, CHK1, and Rad51. *PLoS One,* 2013, 8, e79106.

[63] Govindaraj, C; Tan, P; Walker, P; Wei, A; Spencer, A; Plebanski, M. Reducing TNF receptor 2+ regulatory T cells via the combined action of azacitidine and the HDAC inhibitor, panobinostat for clinical benefit in acute myeloid leukemia patients. *Clin. Cancer Res*., 2014, 20, 724-735.

[64] Novotny-Diermayr, V; Sausgruber, N; Loh, YK; Pasha, MK; Jayaraman, R; Hentze, H; Yong, WP; Goh, BC; Toh, HC; Ethirajulu, K; Zhu, J; Wood, JM. Pharmacodynamic evaluation of the target efficacy of SB939, an oral HDAC inhibitor with selectivity for tumor tissue. *Mol. Cancer Ther*., 2011, 10, 1207-1217.

[65] Bose, P; Grant, S. Orphan drug designation for pracinostat, volasertib and alvocidib in AML. *Leuk. Res.,* 2014, 38, 862-865.

[66] Montalban-Bravo, G; Garcia-Manero, G. Novel drugs for older patients with acute myeloid leukemia. *Leukemia,* 2014; doi: 10.1038/leu.2014.244.

[67] Xu, Y; Voelter-Mahlknecht S; Mahlknecht U. The histone deacetylase inhibitor suberoylanilide hydroxamic acid down-regulates expression levels of Bcr-abl, c-Myc and HDAC3 in chronic myeloid leukemia cell lines. *Int. J. Mol. Med*., 2005, 15, 169-172.

[68] Nimmanapalli, R; Fuino, L; Bali, P; Gasparetto, M; Glozak, M; Tao, J; Moscinski, L; Smith, C; Wu, J; Jove, R; Atadja, P; Bhalla, K. Histone deacetylase inhibitor LAQ824 both lowers expression and promotes proteasomal degradation of Bcr-Abl and induces apoptosis of imatinib mesylate-sensitive or -refractory chronic myelogenous leukemia-blast crisis cells. *Cancer Res.*, 2003, 63, 5126-5135.

[69] Okabe, S; Tauchi, T; Kimura, S; Maekawa, T; Kitahara, T; Tanaka, Y; Ohyashiki, K. Combining the ABL1 kinase inhibitor ponatinib and the histone deacetylase inhibitor vorinostat: a potential treatment for BCR-ABL-positive leukemia. *PLoS One,* 2014, 9, e89080.

[70] Okabe, S; Tauchi, T; Tanaka, Y; Kimura, S; Maekawa, T; Ohyashiki, K. Activity of histone deacetylase inhibitors and an Aurora kinase inhibitor in BCR-ABL-expressing leukemia cells: Combination of HDAC and Aurora inhibitors in BCR-ABL-expressing cells. *Cancer Cell Int.*, 2013, 13, 32.

[71] Mithraprabhu, S; Grigoriadis, G; Khong, T; Spencer, A. Deactylase inhibition in myeloproliferative neoplasms. *Invest. New Drugs,* 2010, 28 (Suppl 1), S50-57.

[72] Rambaldi, A; Dellacasa, CM; Finazzi, G; Carobbio, A; Ferrari, ML; Guglielmelli, P; Gattoni, E; Salmoiraghi, S; Finazzi, MC; Di Tollo, S; D'Urzo, C; Vannucchi, AM; Barosi, G; Barbui, T. A pilot study of the Histone-Deacetylase inhibitor Givinostat in patients with JAK2V617F positive chronic myeloproliferative neoplasms. *Br. J. Haematol.*, 2010, 150, 446-455.

[73] Verstovsek, S; Komrokji, RS. Novel and emerging therapies for the treatment of polycythemia vera. *Expert Rev. Hematol.*, 2014, 29, 1-13.

[74] Mascarenhas, J; Lu, M; Li, T; Petersen, B; Hochman, T; Najfeld, V; Goldberg, JD; Hoffman, R. A phase I study of panobinostat (LBH589) in patients with primary myelofibrosis (PMF) and post-polycythaemia vera/essential thrombocythaemia myelofibrosis (post-PV/ET MF). *Br. J. Haematol.*, 2013, 161, 68-75.

[75] DeAngelo, DJ; Mesa, RA; Fiskus, W; Tefferi, A; Paley, C; Wadleigh, M; Ritchie, EK; Snyder, DS; Begna, K; Ganguly, S; Ondovik, MS; Rine, J; Bhalla, KN. Phase II trial of panobinostat, an oral pan-deacetylase inhibitor in patients with primary myelofibrosis, post-essential thrombocythaemia, and post-polycythaemia vera myelofibrosis. *Br. J. Haematol.*, 2013, 162, 326-335.

[76] Andersen, CL; Mortensen, NB; Klausen, TW; Vestergaard, H; Bjerrum, OW; Hasselbalch, HC. A phase II study of vorinostat (MK-0683) in

patients with primary myelofibrosis and post-polycythemia vera myelofibrosis. *Haematologica,* 2014, 99, e5-7.

[77] Sutheesophon K, Kobayashi Y, Takatoku MA, Ozawa K, Kano Y, Ishii H, Furukawa Y. Histone deacetylase inhibitor depsipeptide (FK228) induces apoptosis in leukemic cells by facilitating mitochondrial translocation of Bax, which is enhanced by the proteasome inhibitor bortezomib. *Acta Haematol.* 2006, 115, 78-90.

[78] Fuchs O, Provaznikova D, Marinov I, Kuzelova K, Spicka I. Antiproliferative and proapoptotic effects of proteasome inhibitors and their combination withhistone deacetylase inhibitors on leukemia cells. *Cardiovasc. Hematol. Dis. Drug Targets* 2009, 9, 62-77.

[79] Nie D, Huang K, Yin S, Li Y, Xie S, Ma L, Wang X, Wu Y, Xiao J. Synergistic/additive interaction of valproic acid with bortezomib on proliferation and apoptosis of acute myeloid leukemia cells. *Leuk. Lymphoma* 2012, 53, 2487-2495.

In: Histone Deacetylase Inhibitors (HDIs) ISBN: 978-1-63463-835-7
Editor: Beverly D. Carson

Chapter 4

HISTONE DEACETYLASE INHIBITORS FOR BREAST CANCER: DRIVING OUT OF STEMNESS

Marion A. Salvador[1,2,3,4], Daniel Birnbaum[1,2,3,4], Emmanuelle Charafe-Jauffret[1,2,3,4] and Christophe Ginestier[1,2,3,4]

[1]Inserm, CRCM, Laboratoire d'Oncologie Moléculaire, Marseille, France
[2]Institut Paoli-Calmettes, Département de Biopathologie, Marseille, France
[3]Aix Marseille Université, Marseille, France
[4]CNRS, CRCM, Marseille, France

ABSTRACT

Breast tumors are believed to be organized in a cellular hierarchy with a population of cancer stem cell (CSC) driving cancer progression and resistance to conventional treatment. The discovery of CSCs provides an explanation for why cancer may be so difficult to cure, and suggests new therapeutic strategies. If these cells are the tumor root, then they are the cells to be killed. CSCs retain key stem cell properties, including self-renewal (which initiates and drives tumorigenesis) and differentiation (albeit aberrant, which contributes to cellular heterogeneity). These last months several reports suggest that HDAC inhibitors can be used to drive

CSCs out of their stemness state through dysregulation of the self-renewal/differentiation balance. Using HDAC inhibitors as a differentiation therapy to treat breast cancers is a promising therapeutic approach to eradicate the breast CSC pool and improve patients care.

COMMENTARY

The intracellular and functional heterogeneity that is observed in breast cancers has been attributed to a specific population of cancer cells, the cancer stem cells (CSC). It has been demonstrated that breast CSCs are responsible for tumor initiation and tumor maintenance locally (tumorigenicity) and for spreading (metastasis) [1]. Conventional therapies, such as chemotherapy or radiotherapy, are unable to eradicate breast CSCs; this failure could explain resistance and relapse of breast cancers. The discovery of CSCs provides an explanation for why cancer may be so difficult to cure, and suggests new therapeutic strategies. Consequently, targeting breast CSCs is critical to improve breast cancer treatment. To design efficient therapeutic strategies targeting CSCs it is crucial to target specific key pathways regulating CSC survival and self-renewal. Several master pathways (Hedgehog, NOTCH, and AKT/WNT/β-catenin signaling) commonly involved in self-renewal of embryonic and adult stem cells are deregulated in CSCs and induce an expansion of this population. A number of agents targeting these pathways are being tested preclinically. Aside of these targeted anti-CSC therapies, another strategy is to drive CSCs out of their stemness state. This latter strategy is called differentiation therapy.

Differentiation therapy using retinoids is successfully used to cure acute promyelocytic leukemia (APL). In APL, the oncogenic fusion protein Promyelocytic Leukemia-Retinoic Acid Receptor α (PML-RARα) binds a histone deacetylase-corepressor complex that prevents transcription of retinoids target genes. Downregulation of the retinoid pathway blocks the differentiation of leukemic progenitors that accumulate. All-trans retinoic acid (ATRA) treatment is able to restore blasts differentiation [2]. Interestingly, a similar approach has been used in breast cancer models suggesting that the self-renewal/differentiation balance can be modulated in breast CSCs [3].

Differentiation therapy aims at disturbing the self-renewal/differentiation balance of CSCs in favor of differentiation. Changing cell fate implies to epigenetically modulate the transcription of self-renewal and differentiation programs. This cellular switch is achieved by regulating the transcription accessibility of coregulated target genes. The acetylation level of histones is a critical coordinator of chromatin condensation and therefore of transcription accessibility. Histone deacetylases (HDAC) are deregulated in most cancers and interact with chromatin modifiers playing thereby a role in tumorigenesis. Thus, epidrugs such as Histone deacetylase inhibitors (HDACis) appear to be excellent candidates for differentiation therapy.

Pioneering studies have shown that HDACis have antiproliferative and apoptotic effects on breast cancers and metastasis [4]. The first observations of breast cancer differentiation were done more than ten years ago by showing morphological and functional changes in breast cancer cell lines [5]. However, it is only recently that two studies have demonstrated that HDACis are able to induce differentiation of breast CSCs [6] and that differentiated cells lose their metastatic potential [7].

Salvador et al. have screened 16 breast cancer cell lines for sensitivity to a new pan-HDACi (abexinostat) and found that 9 out of 16 responded to low-dose treatment. In these low-dose sensitive models they demonstrated that the CSC population decreased after HDACi treatment *in vitro* and *in vivo* using patient-derived xenografts (PDX). The decrease of the tumorigenic CSC population was related to the induction of luminal markers of differentiation, which mimicked a reverse Epithelial-to-Mesenchymal transition (EMT). The EMT program has been identified as a critical regulator of CSCs self-renewal and contributes to confer the metastatic potential of the CSC population [8].

Rhodes et al. have recently reported that HDACis prevent metastasis formation through the inhibition of master regulators of EMT in breast cancer cell lines. They showed that panobinostat inhibited EMT-associated genes (Vimentin, ZEB1, ZEB2) whereas epithelial cadherin (CDH1) was induced. Migration and invasion of treated cells were decreased, and when injected into immunocompromised mice, the number of brain and lung metastases was reduced. Reciprocally, surexpression of the ZEB2 transcription factor reversed the benefits of the panobinostat treatment.

These two recent studies strongly suggest that HDAC inhibition can be considered as a differentiation therapy for breast cancer due to its ability to push CSCs out stemness. If first clinical trials using HDACis in breast cancers were disappointing due to a high toxicity and a moderate effect on tumor shrinkage, we can expect that new HDACis may present a lower toxicity with a direct effect on the tumorigenic cell population. Based on the recent studies, we can now propose a rationale for combination therapy using HDACis and conventional treatments. HDACis would induce breast CSC differentiation and newly differentiated cells could be eradicated with conventional treatments as mere tumor bulk cells (Figure 1). Interestingly, one direct application of breast tumor differentiation seems to be a sensitization to hormone therapy. Functional re-expression of estrogen receptor has been achieved in triple-negative cell lines treated by HDACi due to an inhibition of the Twist/HDAC complex [9]. This has led to the initiation of several clinical trials combining HDACis with anti-estrogen therapy [10]. Interestingly, HDACis also reverse acquired-resistance to hormonal therapy in advanced and metastatic breast cancers [11].

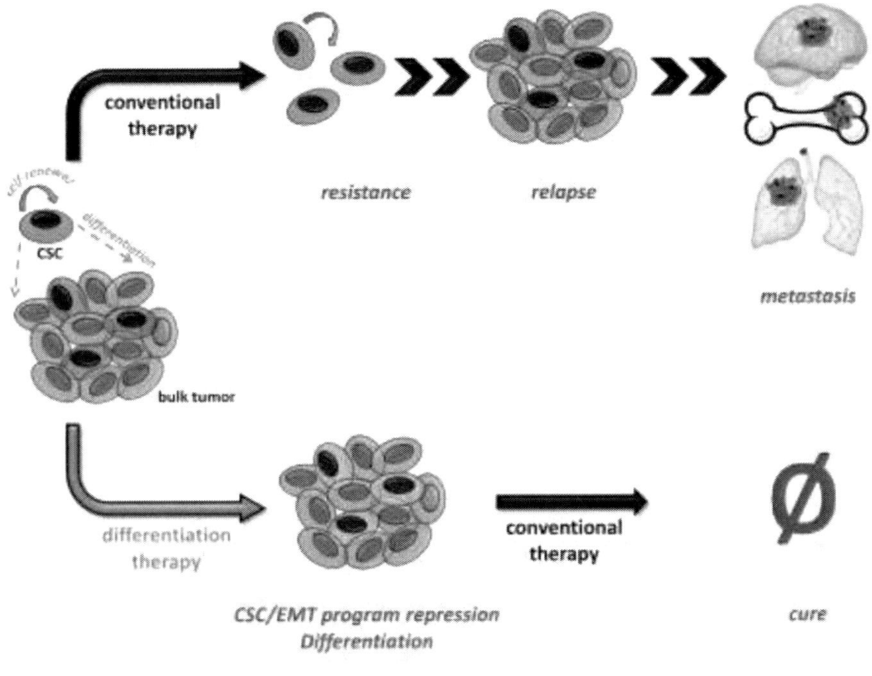

Figure 1. Differentiation therapy for targeting breast cancer stem cells (CSC). Conventional therapies such as chemotherapy, radiotherapy or hormonal therapy are effective for elimination of breast bulk tumor but spare breast cancer stem cells (CSC). CSCs are then able to replenish breast tumor which leads to relapse of the disease and metastasis formation. Differentiating agents such as HDACis would drive out self-renewal/epithelial-to-mesenchymal (EMT) properties and push cell differentiation, thereafter these newly differentiated cells could be sensitized by conventional therapies.

Furthermore, this therapeutic approach can probably be generalized to other epidrugs such as DNA methyltransferase inhibitors. Tsai and colleagues have described a similar phenomenon using decitabine and azacitidine, which induced an antitumor "memory" response, including inhibition of the CSC population [12].

In conclusion, if differentiation therapy has long been restricted to hematologic disease, the development of new epidrugs such as HDACis offers new perspectives for the targeting of CSCs in solid tumors.

REFERENCES

[1] Kreso, A; Dick, JE. Evolution of the cancer stem cell model. *Cell Stem Cell,* 2014 14, 275-91.

[2] Huang, ME; et al. Use of all-trans retinoic acid in the treatment of acute promyelocytic leukemia. *Blood,* 1988 72, 567-72.

[3] Ginestier, C; et al. Retinoid signaling regulates breast cancer stem cell differentiation. *Cell Cycle*, 2009 8, 3297-302.

[4] Palmieri, D; et al. Vorinostat inhibits brain metastatic colonization in a model of triple-negative breast cancer and induces DNA double-strand breaks. *Clinical Cancer Research,* 2009 15, 6148-57.

[5] Munster, PN; et al. The histone deacetylase inhibitor suberoylanilide hydroxamic acid induces differentiation of human breast cancer cells. *Cancer Research,* 2001 61, 8492-7.

[6] Salvador, MA; et al. The histone deacetylase inhibitor abexinostat induces cancer stem cells differentiation in breast cancer with low Xist expression. *Clinical Cancer Research*, 2013 19, 6520-31.

[7] Rhodes, LV; et al. Suppression of triple-negative breast cancer metastasis by pan-DAC inhibitor panobinostat via inhibition of ZEB family of EMT master regulators. *Breast Cancer Research Treatment*, 2014 145, 593-604.

[8] Mani, SA; et al. The epithelial-mesenchymal transition generates cells with properties of stem cells. *Cell,* 2008 133, 704-15.

[9] Vesuna, F; et al. Twist contributes to hormone resistance in breast cancer by downregulating estrogen receptor-α. *Oncogene,* 2012 31, 3223-34.

[10] Thomas, S; et al. Histone deacetylase inhibitor induced modulation of anti-estrogen therapy. *Cancer Letter,* 2009 280, 184-91.

[11] Munster, PN; et al. A phase II study of the histone deacetylase inhibitor vorinostat combined with tamoxifen for the treatment of patients with hormone therapy-resistant breast cancer. *Breast Journal Cancer,* 2011 104, 1828-35.

[12] Tsai, HC; et al. Transient low doses of DNA-demethylating agents exert durable antitumor effects on hematological and epithelial tumor cells. *Cancer Cell,* 2012 21, 430-46.

INDEX

A

B

C

D

E

I

K

L

M

N

O

P

Q

R

S

T

U

V

W

X

Y

Z